MW01104435

Other titles in the series

LATE-BREAKING
AMAZING STORIES™

PLASTIC SURGERY
GONE WRONG

Tragic consequences in the search for beauty

by Melanie Jones

Altitude Publishing

PUBLISHED BY ALTITUDE PUBLISHING LTD.
1500 Railway Avenue, Canmore, Alberta T1W 1P6
www.amazingstoriesbooks.com
1-800-957-6888

Extreme care has been taken to ensure that the information contained in this book is accurate and up to date at the time of printing. However, neither the author nor the publisher is responsible for errors, omissions, loss of income or anything else that may result from the information contained in this book.

Publisher	Stephen Hutchings
Associate Publisher	Kara Turner
Canadian Editor	Rennay Craats
U.S. Editor	Julian S. Martin
Fact Checker	Andy Sayers
Charts	Scott Dutton

We acknowledge the financial support of the Government of Canada through the Book Publishing Industry Development Program (BPIDP) for our publishing activities.

ALTITUDE GREENTREE PROGRAM
Altitude Publishing will plant twice as many trees as were used in the manufacturing of this product.

In order to make this book as universal as possible, all currency is shown in US dollars.

Cataloging in Publication Data
Jones, Melanie
   Plastic surgery gone wrong / Melanie Jones.

(Late breaking amazing stories)
1-55265-302-1 (American mass market edition)
1-55439-505-4 (Canadian mass market edition)

   1. Surgery, Plastic--Popular works. 2. Surgery,
Plastic--Complications--Popular works. I. Title. II. Series.

RD119.J64 2005   617.9'5   C2005-905270-8

In Canada, Amazing Stories® is a registered trademark of Altitude Publishing Canada Ltd. An application for the same trademark is pending in the U.S.

Printed and bound in Canada by Friesens
2 4 6 8 9 7 5 3 1

"Some patients put more time into choosing a pair of shoes than they do choosing a plastic surgeon."

Dr. Teresa Ghazoul, plastic surgeon

CONTENTS

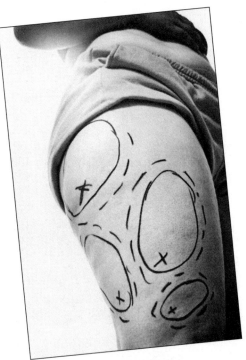

A woman's thigh marked up for
liposuction. (For the story on the
dangers of liposuction see page 76.)

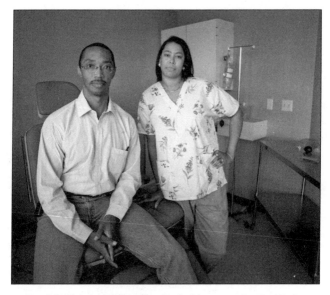

Patrick Chavis, M.D., left, sits in his operating room in his Lynwood, California, office with his nurse Carlitha Allen. This photograph is dated August 1997. (For more on the Patrick Chavis story see page 79.)

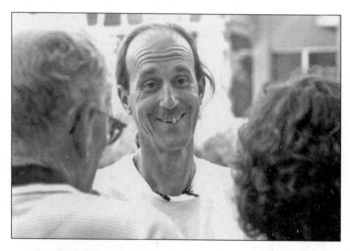

Ray Krone, center, smiles at his mother and stepfather on his release from Arizona's Florence Prison in April 2002. Krone was imprisoned for 10 years for a crime he did not commit. (See facing page.)

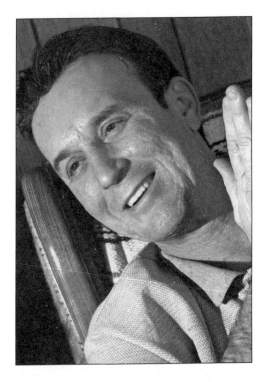

The same Ray Krone photographed February 11,
2005, following his dramatic transformation on ABC's
"Extreme Makeover." Family and friends who saw the
new Ray for the first time on January 19, 2005,
were amazed. (For more on Ray Krone
story see page 48.)

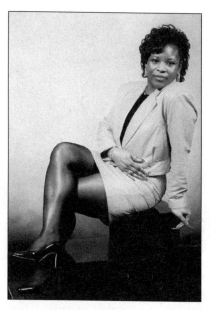

An undated photograph of Tammaria Cotton, a
healthy, married mother from Los Angeles who died
following liposuction surgery in 1996. (For more
on the tragic story of Tammaria Cotton see page 83.)

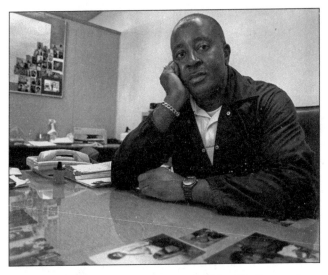

Jimmy Cotton, with photographs of his wife, Tammaria
(opposite), who died after liposuction surgery.
(For more on the tragic story of Tammaria Cotton
see page 83.)

CHAPTER 1

Introducing Plastic Surgery

She was a diabetic wife and mother of two, and she was 200 pounds overweight. She'd had her insulin under control for a couple of years now, but no matter what she did, she couldn't take off the weight. She'd tried dieting and even had her stomach stapled, but nothing had worked. She'd read about bariatric or weight loss surgery before. It involved extensive liposuction and then a full body lift to tighten the excess, baggy skin afterward. More than 50,000 people had it done in 2003. She figured she'd been through enough with her diabetes; it was time to treat herself to looking better. She went in for the several-hour procedure with high hopes, even though her husband was leery. After being put to sleep, a cocktail of local anesthetic and another drug to stop the bleeding were flushed under her skin. Then, using a thin tube, the surgeon sucked out several pounds of fat from her legs, abdomen, buttocks, back, and arms. She woke up groggy and in terrible pain. Within several hours, the pain hadn't abated, and now bloody fluid was seeping out of her 11 incisions. The pain in her legs wouldn't lessen and the bruising over the next few weeks was horrible. Eventually, her legs began turning black. She went to the hospital, and a doctor told her that her legs were severely infected and gangrenous. The skin on her legs was essentially dying. They would have to amputate. Two months after going in for plastic surgery to improve her looks, she was in a wheelchair with both legs cut off above the knee.

To many people, plastic or cosmetic surgery has become the next quick-fix to weight problems or low self-esteem. It has become ubiquitous, with many Hollywood stars going under the knife to perfect their already gorgeous bodies and faces. Now, more and more "regular" people are opting for surgery to combat the signs of aging with facelifts, breast augmentation, Botox®, and liposuction. What most people don't realize are the incredible risks of surgery for the sake of vanity. A surgery is only as good as the surgeon performing it, and doctors' credentials and skills are easily overlooked, or worse, false. As well, general anesthesia can lead to blood clots and heart failure under even the best circumstances. And there are all-too-common post-surgery effects such as serious infection, uneven healing, unexpected scarring, and sometimes constant pain. It turns out that plastic surgery is not the quick fix it's marketed to be.

It has been suggested that cosmetic surgery isn't even medicine—as medicine is defined as the practice of diagnosing and treating disease or injury. It is an aesthetic service more akin to a spa. Some also say that it is the "Surgery of the Psyche," a sort of surgical psychiatry that helps patients improve their self-esteem. Regardless, cosmetic surgery's place in the grey areas between medicine and aesthetics, where health insurance stops and board certification begins, makes it one of the most hotly debated surgical practices of the day.

CHAPTER 2

The Issue

Marilyn Monroe was a size 12. She was revered as one of the most beautiful women in the world, and indeed in history. By today's standards, however, Marilyn was positively fat. Hollywood and the news media have tracked and influenced the ever-shifting concept of beauty for the last hundred years, impacting the general population in unprecedented ways. It is perhaps a circular argument as to whether media dictate the fashion or simply report it, but regardless, the influence of mass media on the beauty industry is almost a given. Trends in fashion, makeup, and hairstyles have now become eclipsed by more permanent forms of self-improvement: plastic and cosmetic surgery and non-surgical procedures such as Botox®. Now a multi-billion dollar industry in North America, cosmetic procedures have exploded in popularity over the past 10 years with huge growth in the last 5. In 1997, there were 2.1 million cosmetic procedures performed per year; by 2003, the numbers had jumped to 8.3 million. That's almost a 300 percent increase. There were 9.2 million surgical procedures in 2004 rising to 11.9 million when including non-surgical procedures like Botox®. Despite an economic downturn, Americans spent $8.4 billion on cosmetic surgery in 2004.

Hollywood and the American film and television industry have influenced the boom in the breast business in several ways. American films present models and actors as perfect, almost superhuman beings with ideal physical forms, from long legs to pearl-white smiles. The growth of the movie industry shows that the general population is buying into the ideal. Hollywood films create an element of fantasy, of escapism, and the beautiful people are a means to that end. As well, the news media are preoccupied with the stars' personal lives. Magazines such as *People* and *US Weekly* track the comings and goings of Hollywood celebrities, imploring readers to be fascinated with where Julia Roberts buys groceries and how Goldie Hawn really looks in a bikini.

The cult of celebrity has led to a continent-wide obsession with film and music stars who, as a group, only make up a tiny portion of the population. In fact, a 2003 study conducted by psychologists at the University of Florida and Southern Illinois University concluded that about one-third of Americans suffer from

Celebrity Worship Syndrome. Behaviors of the syndrome range from a rather benign group comprising 20 percent of the population that follows celebrity news for social purposes. A second group, 10 percent of the population, develops an intense (if imagined) relationship with a star. The third and scariest group, roughly one percent of the population, displays borderline pathological behavior. Some people who fall into this category also look to plastic surgery, modeling their own facial features after celebrities'. Interestingly, MTV recently launched a reality television show called *I Want a Famous Face*. The program follows young people who undergo plastic surgery in order to look like their favorite stars: more evidence that "normal" people can't measure up on their own.

The average American woman is 5 feet 5 inches tall and weighs 144 pounds. The average American model is 5 feet 11 inches tall and weighs 117 pounds. Models and actors represent a minute sliver of humanity, employed for their considerable talents and gifts, not the least of which is their physical attractiveness. A world-wide obsession with beauty has focused its gaze on Hollywood, and Hollywood has responded by showing us actresses who keep getting thinner while their breasts keep getting bigger and actors with heads full of thick hair and torsos full of well-defined muscles. The great irony of it all is the impossible standards these images create. For example, breasts are largely composed of fat. If a woman loses weight, her breasts tend to get smaller. Achieving Hollywood's standard of a stick-thin body with DD-cup breasts is virtually impossible without the aid of surgery. Large and defined muscles in men are usually achieved by hard work at the gym, but some do it through the use of anabolic steroids, liposuction, or both. California Governor and former action hero, Arnold Schwarzenegger openly admits to steroid use to create his hulking look. A full 10 percent of all liposuction procedures done in 2004 were performed on men, more than 32,000 procedures. More than 43,000 hair transplants were done as well.

Some of Hollywood's elite are open about their many surgical alterations. Cher has spoken publicly about her facelifts and breast augmentation (although she is more hush-hush about her liposuction) and even refers to herself as the plastic surgery "poster girl." Joan Rivers is open about her many facelifts and encourages other stars to talk about it as well. But most celebrities are incredibly close-lipped about their cosmetic histories, and many stars who you wouldn't expect have had work done. Uma Thurman has had a nose job, Julia Roberts a breast augmentation, Tara Reid breast augmentation and liposuction, and even young star Natalie Portman has had nose work done.

The Aging Face of America

Hollywood isn't the only cause of the "plastics explosion." The population is aging as baby boomers get older. This is the generation that, in many ways, has made North American society what it is today. The boomers invented the computer, The Gap, and bumped the divorce rate up to 49 percent in the United States (43 percent in Canada), according to *Divorce Magazine*. At 90 million strong, they are the single most influential economic group in North America. According to a report on CBS news, this generation now accounts for an incredible one trillion dollars in annual income. To put it simply, they *are* the economy.

BABY BOOMERS

Sociologists most commonly define baby boomers as those born between 1946 and 1964. There are about 76 million boomers in the U.S. The U.S. and Canada combined have 90 million.

Health care advances over the past hundred years mean we as a population are living longer, healthier lives. As a result, many people don't *feel* old and therefore don't want to look it either. As the average age rises steadily, so does the impulse to combat the signs of aging. In fact, one of the characteristics of the baby boomers is a fear of getting old. Another characteristic of this demographic group is the desire to have it all and have it all right now and having the money to get it.

Anti-aging medicine is based on the notion that aging is a treatable condition, a radically new idea. Anti-aging medicine is an extension of preventative health care—a multidisciplinary approach aimed at detecting, preventing, and reversing age-related diseases such as cancer, diabetes, and Alzheimer's. But it's more than medicine. The anti-aging movement has turned into a multi-billion dollar industry that includes yoga and Pilates classes, skincare regimens, meditation workshops, vitamins and supplements, massage therapy, weight loss programs, spa treatments, and cosmetic surgery. The diet, nutrition, and personal care industries alone are now estimated to be a $56-billion annual market. This is expected to double over the next five years.

So the increase in cosmetic surgery could

be, rather simplistically, linked to the baby boomers. In 2005, this segment of the population was between 41 and 59 years old. In 1997, when the plastic surgery statistics began their drastic increase from 2.1 million procedures per year to the current level of more than 12 million, they were 33 to 51 years old. In other words, they were old enough to see the effects of aging and they were going to do something about it. But surgery doesn't always go according to plan.

Lynn Dugan was 55 years old, and her aging skin was beginning to remind her of her mother. Hoping to erase a few years from her face, she decided to try a facelift. She never imagined things could go as wrong as they did. Lynn admits she made a few mistakes. She found an attractive advertisement in the *Yellow Pages*, but didn't thoroughly check the doctor's credentials (his license was in fact suspended). From the first visit with her surgeon, things were amiss. She says the doctor didn't take her blood pressure or any blood tests before the procedure. He gave Lynn a prescription for antibiotics to take following her surgery, but when they didn't agree with her, he gave her no instructions other than to discontinue them. Lynn learned later that the surgeon's 22-year-old daughter (who had no training in medicine) assisted in her surgery.

The night of her facelift, Lynn went home. She developed a fever and went to bed. By the following week, she still had chills and a fever. She was also weak and her thinking was "fuzzy." She returned to the doctor's office, this time in a wheelchair, but he diagnosed her with the flu and sent her home. Her condition did not improve.

Several days later her husband, Doug, took her to the emergency room of a local hospital. There, doctors found pus seeping from her infected incisions. Lynn Dugan was diagnosed with necrotizing fasciitis, or flesh-eating disease, an aggressive illness that can result in amputation, horrible disfigurement, or death.

Lynn was in intensive care for more than

a month and during those 34 days, most of her internal organs began to shut down. Doctors punctured her chest to drain fluid that had built up, and her toes were so badly infected they considered amputating. Later, skin grafts were taken from her legs to replace the necrotized skin on her chest. Well after her frightening ordeal, it would take three more operations to stop the infection, repair the damage, and remove the scars. This certainly wasn't what Lynn Dugan imagined when she entered the surgeon's office.

No Beauty Salon

Many people like Lynn Dugan think of plastic or cosmetic surgery as a simple outpatient procedure in a stylishly decorated downtown clinic. But plastic surgery is not just a trip to the beauty parlor; it is major surgery with all the attendant risks and a few unique complications of its own. Add that to lengthy healing times, bruising, and swelling, and it presents profound challenges for patients and the medical profession alike. In a 1997 study, the American Board of Plastic Surgeons (ABPS) put the risk of serious complications at less than half of one percent. They also said that the risk of death from plastic surgery affected 1 in 57,000 patients. With patients totaling more than 9 million in 2004, that's definitely a statistic to watch.

THE RISKS OF LOOKING BEAUTIFUL

- Scarring
- Nerve damage
- Blood clots
- Infection
- Bleeding
- Rejection of implants or sutures
- Necrotizing fasciitis (flesh-eating disease)
- Bruising and hematoma (blood pooling under the skin)
- Skin necrosis (skin death)
- Capsular contracture in breast implants (extreme scarring around the implant, resulting in misshapen breasts)
- Adverse reactions to anesthesia

Any major surgery comes with inherent risks, most of which are connected to general anesthesia. Use of general anesthetic, where the patient is rendered unconscious, is the highest risk form of sedation or anesthesia with possible complications including airway obstruction, brain damage, nerve damage, heart attack, stroke, and even death. Studies have reported the death rate resulting from general anesthesia at anywhere from 0.0005 deaths per 1,000 cases to a whopping 3.8 per 1,000.

In general, the longer the surgery lasts and the more blood that's lost, the greater becomes the risk of complications. Extended surgeries increase the risk of deep venous thrombosis (DVT). DVT involves the formation of a blood clot in the larger veins of the leg. The clot can interfere with circulation in the area, and it could break off and travel through the bloodstream. The blood clot can lodge in the brain, lungs, or heart, causing severe damage or even death. Other common risks of surgery and surgical recovery are blood clots, which can be fatal, and infection, which in some cases has resulted in amputation of gangrenous body parts. One of the risks specific to plastic surgery is skin necrosis, or skin death. Necrosis occurs when not enough blood is supplied to the tissue. Once it occurs, it is not reversible. Infection occurs in less than one percent of cases, but the more procedures performed at one time, the higher the risk of infection.

Such risks never occurred to Paul Falaschi, a 25-year-old handsome and fit personal trainer in San Francisco. He was acutely self-conscious, though, of a small roll at his waist. So much so, that he decided to undergo liposuction. Apparently embarrassed to admit the truth, Paul told his friends he had kidney stones when he went to St. Francis Memorial Hospital on November 6, 1997. There, a plastic surgeon spent three hours vacuuming fat from his abdomen, buttocks, thighs, and lower back. Four days later, he succumbed to an aggressive blood infection believed to have been a common strain of streptococcus. Paul Falaschi's was the fourth liposuction-related death reported in the United States in 1997.

Liposuction is one of the riskiest, and most

inconsistently reported, cosmetic procedures. One of liposuction's greatest risks is embolism, which occurs when fat enters the blood stream through blood vessels broken during the liposuction and becomes trapped in blood vessels, gathers in the lungs, or travels to the brain. A review of mortality studies published by Dr. Robert Yoho *et al.* reveals some wildly varying numbers. Some studies indicate that the risk of death due to liposuction is as low as 3 deaths for every 100,000 liposuction operations performed. A study of 1,200 board-certified American Society for Aesthetic Plastic Surgery (ASAPS) members reported a significantly higher death rate: 1 in 5,224 procedures. But when this and other liposuction risk-rate studies were independently reviewed by Rockwell and Daane in the *Journal of Aesthetic Plastic Surgery* in 1999, the death rate for liposuction was found to be as high as 1 in 1,000 in some instances.

The fact that many procedures like liposuction are performed in outpatient facilities only serves to compound the risk. In both the United States and Canada, outpatient or ambulatory surgery has become the most popular option for doctors. Unfortunately quality control, which is strictly adhered to in public hospitals, is difficult to regulate in outpatient units. Uncertified surgeons (such as family doctors, dermatologists, and anesthetists) and those unable to perform specific procedures at the hospital where they hold admitting privileges (such as ear, nose, and throat surgeons who wish to do breast and body contour surgery) opened ambulatory centers in record numbers in the 1990s. Surgeries performed in private clinics or surgical facilities are riskier than those done in hospitals, which are better equipped to handle emergencies. In February 1999, physicians in Florida performing office-based procedures were required to begin reporting certain events, including patient deaths and emergency transfers to hospitals. Since the Florida Agency for Health Care Administration began collecting this data,

58 hospital transfers and 19 deaths have been reported.

The Push for Profits

The increased risks associated with private facilities point to one of the major issues affecting cosmetic surgery today: privatized health care. This is where the American and Canadian health care systems drastically diverge. Canadians have a publicly funded health care system to which every citizen has access. For most medically necessary treatments in Canada, no fees are charged; the cost is covered by taxes.

In the United States, however, the delivery of health care is for the most part in the hands of for-profit private enterprise. Most Americans have private health insurance that is often paid for by their employers. If they get sick and require medical treatment, the insurance company pays the bills. A 2003 study published in the *New England Journal of Medicine* says the per-person cost of U.S. health care is $1,059 while in Canada it's $307. The huge difference is mostly due to the added administrative costs of processing payment through scores of insurance companies.

The field of plastic surgery is divided into two types: reconstructive and cosmetic. Reconstructive surgery, such as surgeries for burn or trauma victims, is medically necessary. Reconstructive procedures are covered mainly by commercial or government health insurance. Payment to the surgeon is subject to the insurers' many payment calculation rules and to regional variations. Cosmetic surgery, however, is generally not medically necessary and therefore not covered by most health insurance policies. Fees are established by the surgeon, and payment is generally received up front. The surgeon must pay various overhead costs, such as surgical assistance and administration, but the rest of the fee is profit. Depending on consumer demand and the surgeon's level of output, profits can rocket sky-high. A 2001 survey of salary levels for plastic surgeons revealed a median of $345,000 and a top-range salary of around $567,000. Other studies report up to $2 million per year for some surgeons. Plastic surgeons aren't the top-paid physicians (cardiologists and radiologists are paid more), but the consumer volume demand has huge appeal.

With the advent of managed health care in the U.S. in the 1980s, insurers started reducing the fees paid out to doctors. This had a drastic effect on their incomes and many looked for ways to make up the loss. Elective surgery seemed like the perfect solution. Liposuction courses were offered over a couple of weekends, and the fees from elective procedures went straight to the bottom line.

In September 2004, New Jersey became the first, and so far the only, state to tax plastic surgery. This 6 percent sales tax has been called Vanity Tax and Luxury Tax. Professional plastic surgeons' organizations were outraged, but the rationale was twofold. In the contemporary anti-tax climate, one-off tax initiatives like this are more palatable. The decision was also based on the assumption that if patients have the money for elective plastic surgery, they will be able to afford the tax. Critics called the tax sexist, as about 88 percent of plastic surgery consumers are women. Regardless, the tax is projected to bring in $25 million a year. More and more American states are now exploring the vanity tax option as well. In Canada, any procedure deemed not medically necessary is subject to 7 percent federal sales tax across the country.

The taxman wasn't the first or only one to see the potential financial benefits of the booming cosmetic surgery business. Credit card companies, insurance companies, and lending institutions have capitalized on the trend with the introduction of cosmetic surgery credit cards (used specifically for elective surgery) and special financing plans. As a result, some young women are now hundreds of thousands of dollars in debt before their 30th birthdays.

Licensing, Legislation, and Malpractice

In the United States, any medical doctor can perform plastic surgery. That means a general practitioner, or family doctor, can legally perform facelifts and liposuction without any surgical training. Drawn by the huge income potential, family doctors and even dentists have been performing major surgery with serious consequences. Medical licensing, the minimum requirement to practice medicine, is administered by individual states. It is not specialty-specific and permits a doctor to provide any medical or surgical service he or she desires.

Every medical resource, newspaper, and magazine article urges consumers to seek out "board-certified" plastic surgeons, and with very good reason. Doctors certified by the American Board of Plastic Surgery (ABPS) have graduated from an accredited medical school and have completed at least five years of additional training as a surgeon. This includes a minimum of three years in general surgery and a minimum of two years in plastic surgery. Then, the doctor must successfully complete comprehensive written and oral exams. In Canada, certification comes from the Royal College of Physicians and Surgeons and follows similar requirements. Surgeons must have at least five years of specialized training (after medical school), including at least two years of general surgery and three years of plastic surgery.

In the United States, board certification is a voluntary process. Board-certified surgeons are relatively easy to find: the Internet is rife with lists of them provided by the ABPS and the American Association of Aesthetic Plastic Surgeons. Unfortunately, patients can find plenty of uncertified surgeons as well. Uncertified doctors performing plastic surgery have presented a huge and frightening problem as patients seek out cheaper prices. Uncertified doctors can perform their surgeries in relative secret, as state accreditation bodies cannot possibly keep up with the scourge of bargain basement plastic surgeons.

For many patients, price may be the limiting factor in their choice of surgeon. And even a certified surgeon can make mistakes.

Dr. Geoffrey Keyes, a board-certified plastic surgeon from Los Angeles, has had at least 23 lawsuits filed against him. The surgeon best known for working on Monica Lewinsky's former friend Linda Tripp has been accused of botching surgeries resulting in everything from eyes not fully closing after eyelifts and excessive scarring after facelifts to shifting chin implants. One of his patients, Kay Marchioni, was in her late 50s when she decided to treat herself to an eyelid lift after surviving a bout of skin cancer. After a phone consultation (Kay lives in Chicago), Keyes and Kay agreed on a price of $12,000. She entered the office expecting only work around her eyes. Keyes insisted they agreed on a facelift. Kay received a full facelift and was left with a 2-inch (5 cm) scar on her chin. She also had an uneven hairline, excessive scarring and swelling, numbness in her left leg, and an infection in her ears as a result of blood clots.

When Kay Marchioni went back to complain, she was met with what she described as unbridled hostility. She says that Keyes showed her graphic photographs of a similar procedure while yelling at her not to ever question him. Keyes, of course, denied it all. When Kay saw Linda Tripp on Jay Leno, something clicked. Tripp said that her chin implant had begun to move, and she had seen another surgeon to repair the flaws from Keyes's surgery. Kay started digging. She found 22 other lawsuits filed against Dr. Geoffrey Keyes. This knowledge sparked a crusade that would lead her to spend more than $50,000 of her retirement savings and hundreds of hours in research. As part of her research, Kay met Ana Diaz, a 27-year-old secretary who saw Keyes for breast reduction surgery.

Ana's F-cup breasts were causing her incredible back pain and even causing her spine to curve unnaturally. She went to Dr. Keyes who said he'd reduce her breasts to a C-cup. When she walked out of surgery, they were barely an A. But that wasn't the only reason she sued. Her breasts were not healing properly, and one day in the shower her nipples fell off. Ana was offered a $200,000 settlement, which she declined, and the case went to court. In the courtroom, Keyes's attorneys noted how well Ana was doing since the surgery: she had a new well-paying job as an Allstate insurance agent, a new boyfriend, and had vacationed in Hawaii. Keyes won the judgment.

Kay Marchioni's missionary zeal led her to track down every one of Keyes's former patients who had filed lawsuits, including several who did not want to get involved. She was militant in her approach, exhausting her lawyer, who had agreed to the case despite the less-than-profitable reputation of malpractice suits. Two days before trial, Kay Marchioni's lawyer backed out. She was forced to defend herself. On the first day of trial the judge asked her to call her first witness. "I have no one to call," she said. The case was thrown out of court.

These cases are tragic, but they have served a purpose; they have prompted lawmakers to sit up and take notice of some flaws in the system. For example, monitoring of health care practices is done at a state level and after increases in deaths and disfigurements in various states, lawmakers have tightened the rules. In La Habra, California, in 1997, one patient died after more than 10 hours of plastic surgery, including large-scale liposuction. Both the doctor, William Earle Matory Jr., and the anesthesiologist, Dr. Robert Ken Hoo, were stripped of their medical licenses. In the same year, Patrick Chavis, an obstetrician-gynecologist who had taken a four-day course at the Liposuction Institute of Beverly Hills, was implicated in the death of one patient and the serious harm of two others. A state crackdown in Florida in the late 1990s revealed that 11 out of 12 reported outpatient surgery deaths were during cosmetic procedures. Another report showed that between 2002 and 2004, three out of eight patients who died in Florida had undergone combination liposuction/abdominoplasty (tummy tuck) procedures in an office setting. A fourth death occurred after a liposuction/fat transfer. These deaths, in part, prompted the Florida Board of Medicine to issue a 90-day ban on the combined procedure in February 2004, saying that the combination of procedures increases the risks of blood clots, leading to pulmonary failure. Under the ban, these procedures had to be performed at least 14 days apart and for the first time, doctors were required to submit surgical logs for procedures done in an office over the previous 2-year period. The Board hoped this would help make office surgeries as safe as possible.

Reality TV and The Extreme Makeover Boom

One of the biggest single influences on the field

of modern plastic surgery has been reality television. Reality TV has been a genre for a long time, beginning with the PBS documentary series *An American Family* in 1973. Since then, reality crime shows represented the market with programs including *America's Most Wanted* and *Cops.* But, the genre took on a life of its own at the launch of CBS's *Survivor* in 1999, which followed castaways on a deserted island. From there, reality TV has exploded with a show for almost every subject, from swapping wives to remaking your home or even remaking yourself. The genre that began with one or two shows on major networks now boasts well over 100 shows on every major and specialty network on the airwaves. It was only a matter of time before plastic surgery became part of it.

There are currently at least two plastic surgery-based reality shows and one dramatic series called *Nip/Tuck* on television. Fox Broadcasting's *The Swan* and ABC's *Extreme Makeover* transform shy, plain-looking people with low confidence into new and improved versions of themselves over the course of several weeks through major and multiple plastic surgery procedures, on top of cosmetic dentistry, hair, fashion, makeup, fitness, and diet.

The Swan employs a therapist and a so-called life coach (show founder Nelly Galan) to guide the two "ugly ducklings" through their transformations in each episode. At the end of the episode, only one wins the right to compete in the Swan Pageant at the end of the season. The list of procedures the show's contestants undergo reads like a cosmetic surgery catalog. A 28-year old flight attendant from Maryland named Kelly had a transformation that included an eyebrow lift, lip enhancement, liposuction of her chin, cheeks, back, calves, ankles, thighs, buttocks, and knees, microdermabrasion, collagen treatments for her lips and nose, laser hair removal, LASIK eye surgery, breast augmentation, dental bleaching, root canals, and dental repair. Kelly also ate only 1,200 calories per day, lifted weights, and did cardio workouts twice per day. The result: a complete transformation over the span of a few weeks.

ABC's *Extreme Makeover* is remarkably similar, except that the show's mandate includes men. *Extreme Makeover* prefers to cast people with interesting, poignant, or compelling stories. Past participants have included twin sisters born with cleft palates, mother-daughter duos, and even wrongly-convicted killers. Ray Krone, an Air Force veteran and mailman, spent 10 years in prison and two on death row for a murder he didn't commit. He was convicted of the 1989 murder of a bar waitress in Phoenix. Ray frequented the bar where she worked and didn't think much of her death until the police arrived at his door. Unbeknownst to Ray, the victim had a crush on him and was heard talking about Ray on a number of occasions. This was enough to spark police suspicion after her death.

Known as The Snaggletooth Killer, the only evidence against Ray Krone was the pattern of bite marks on the victim. Ray's crooked front teeth landed him on death row, despite the fact that other evidence pointed police in other directions. Ten years later, DNA evidence proved his innocence and Ray Krone became the 100th person exonerated from a murder conviction. After his release, he worked as a motivational speaker, doing odd jobs on the side. Ten years in prison and the extreme stress of a wrongful conviction had taken their toll on his appearance. He looked aged and defeated, with a receding hair line and sunken chest. His skin was battered by acne scars, and a ratty moustache did nothing to hide the teeth that had literally ruined his life.

Compelled by his story, the producers of *Extreme Makeover* approached 47-year-old Ray Krone. His makeover included rhinoplasty, eyebrow lift, upper and lower eyelid lift, liposuction of his chin, laser resurfacing, acne scar excision, hair transplant, hair restoration, LASIK eye surgery, photo facial, sonopeel (which uses water to remove dead skin), oxygen facial, filler to acne scars and nasal labial folds, muscle relaxer to forehead, 4 tooth extractions, 4 permanent tooth implants, 17 porcelain crowns and veneers, and tooth whitening. Ray's lawyer estimated the value of these treatments at over $200,000. After it all, the new, improved Ray Krone looked nothing like the man who was convicted, retried, convicted again, sent to death row, and ultimately cleared of murder.

Stories like Ray Krone's highlight the positive effects plastic surgery has on people. But it, like the shows themselves, is extreme. Participants on plastic surgery reality shows are rigorously screened for physical and psychological health before undergoing multiple operations. Their televised transformations appear quick and comprehensive, and the shows make it look easy. All of the procedures in Ray's makeover took place over only two months—a potentially dangerous undertaking. Many plastic surgeons warn, "Do not try this yourself."

Reality shows trivialize cosmetic surgery. They tend to distort public perceptions about the practice, its possibilities, and its safety. Television show participants are subjected to multiple procedures in one surgical experience—an incredibly risky endeavor. The state of Florida's medical board banned the double procedure of liposuction and tummy tuck in 2004 for this very reason. The longer the surgery takes, the greater the risk of complications becomes. Since the release of these television programs, plastic surgeons have been inundated with patients requesting to be made over overnight. Most procedures take weeks, even months, to heal, and patients almost always look worse before they look better. But much of the bruising, swelling, and post-surgery pain ends up on reality television's cutting room floor. Some surgeons have taken advantage of the booming business this television exposure has created; others are appalled by it. "This is a major surgical procedure, not a hairdo," Adam Searle, president of the British Association of Aesthetic Plastic Surgery (BAAPS) has said. According to him, and many other surgeons, the public is beginning to see cosmetic surgery as a trip to the salon.

This line is further blurred with the advent of so-called medispas, where customers can receive Botox® injections along with their pedicures. In fact, Botox®, which uses the botulism toxin to paralyze the musculature of the face and smooth out lines, is marketed as a cosmetic. Some plastic surgeons have even blended their practices with full-service spas, providing anything from a facial to a facelift.

Plastoholics and Body Dysmorphic Disorder

Hope Donahue was a pretty girl from a well-off Los Angeles family. When she was 22 years old, she paid for her first cosmetic surgery operation, a nose job, with her credit cards. The next year, she had her first facelift. By the age of 27.

she'd had seven surgeries. Her parents were shocked with what they called her "self-mutilation." They stopped giving her money and asked her to leave the family home so they wouldn't have to see her downward spiral into a horrible obsession with plastic surgery. Hope didn't get a regular day job, though. In order to fuel her addiction, she began stealing. She posed nude in order to make money. She says she hit bottom the day she found herself in an S&M photographer's studio. She walked out of the studio and started therapy.

In an appearance on Oprah, Hope referred to herself as "a recovering addict." She had her last surgery 10 years ago to remove her breast implants but confesses to such procedures as Botox® and collagen injections since then. She told Oprah Winfrey that each time she "falls off the wagon," she feels like she's failed. She has scheduled and then canceled four nose job surgeries, and like many addicts, recovery is a daily battle. She is the author of a book called

Beautiful Stranger, a tell-all memoir of her battle with body dysmorphic disorder, or BDD.

Body dysmorphic disorder isn't a new phenomenon, but one that has come out of the closet in part because of its relationship with plastic surgery. BDD is an excessive preoccupation with a real or imagined defect in a person's physical appearance. People with BDD have a distorted or exaggerated view of how they look and are obsessed with perceived flaws, such as a deformed nose or acne. They often think of themselves as ugly or disfigured. People with the disorder commonly have problems controlling negative thoughts about their appearance, even when reassured by others that they look fine. BDD affects between one and two percent of the North American population, and as many as half of these sufferers turn to plastic surgery or dermatological treatments to correct their perceived defects. The American Academy of Cosmetic Surgery estimates that two percent of cosmetic surgery patients have BDD.

Body dysmorphic disorder is a debilitating problem that causes people excessive anxiety and distress, often leading to social isolation and impairing their performance at school or work. People with BDD may find it difficult to meet new people or make friends because they believe they will be judged as ugly. People with BDD repeatedly check themselves in mirrors, wear bulky clothing or excessive makeup to hide an offending body part, touch or pick at themselves obsessively, and seek constant reassurance that they look "normal." People with severe BDD may drop out of school, quit their jobs, or avoid leaving their homes. In the most severe cases, people with BDD may attempt suicide or become violent toward others. There are at least two reported cases of plastic surgery patients with BDD whose surgeries led to disaster. Theresa Mary Ramirez shot and killed her plastic surgeon after receiving her 13th breast surgery. Beryl Challis was unhappy with her facelift and shot her doctor with a .38

caliber handgun before later turning the gun on herself.

BDD has also been linked to Obsessive Compulsive Disorder (OCD) because of symptoms such as constantly checking or picking at the skin, and many BDD sufferers also experience severe depression. As many men as women are affected by this disorder, with men frequently thinking their muscles are too small or that their build is inadequate. They will often take steroids and exercise excessively to try and correct these imagined or exaggerated defects.

Even though up to half of BDD sufferers

BDD HELP GROUPS

- www.bddcentral.com is a forum for information and help for people with BDD
- National Association of Anorexia Nervosa and Associated Disorders, hotline for referral in your area: 1-847-831-3438
- www.mental-health-today.com has an online BDD forum, plus contact numbers for support or crisis
- Most cities and towns will have some kind of support group for body image problems. Contact your local mental health organization to be put in touch with a local BDD resource.

seek cosmetic surgery to deal with their perceived flaws, surgery may have the opposite effect of making the symptoms worse. Patients may undergo a rhinoplasty and either not be satisfied with the results or transfer their dissatisfaction to another body part. Fundamentally, the problem involves distorted body image and a tendency to obsess and worry as opposed to a real, physical deformity. The unfortunate result is something akin to an addiction to plastic surgery. A patient will keep coming back to the surgeon, asking for more and more work done on the same part. If refused treatment, he or she will simply try another surgeon. But nothing any surgeon does will fix the problems—problems that don't physically exist.

A study published in 2000 found that some BDD sufferers take matters into their own hands. The study found that 9 out of 25 patients performed their own do-it-yourself plastic surgery in order to alter their appearance. One man, who believed that his skin was too loose, used a staple gun on both sides of his face to try to keep his skin taut. The staples fell out after 10 minutes and he narrowly missed damaging his facial nerve. Another woman who wanted liposuction but could not afford it used a knife to cut her thighs and attempted to squeeze out the fat.

One of the most famous plastoholics is pop singer/songwriter Michael Jackson. Jackson is extremely close-mouthed about his cosmetic surgery, admitting to only two rhinoplasty surgeries. But over the years, the public has watched as his face and skin tone have changed drastically. The singer's formerly wide nose has been altered several times. It was rumored at one stage that his now razor-thin nose had fallen off. (Perhaps for this reason, the pop singer wore a transparent bandage over the tip of his nose for most of his 2005 child-molestation trial.) While this seems outlandish, it is an actual hazard of excessive plastic surgery. Patients are warned that their noses may collapse with too much surgical work, but many people do it anyway. Another well-known side effect of plastic surgery is skin necrosis, in which lack of blood flow causes flesh to simply fall off.

Jackson's cheek-bones and jawline have also become more pro-nounced over the years, a cleft chin appeared in the early 1990s, and his eyebrows are unnatu-rally high. Moreover, his skin tone changed from a cocoa brown to a uniform shade of white. The singer blames a skin condi-tion called vitiligo, in

ASPS BRIEFING PAPERS

The American Society of Plastic Surgeons (ASPS) has released two briefing papers informing and warning the general public about issues of concern related to plastic and cosmetic surgery.

The first warning was released in August 2004 concerning the growing trend of plastic surgery in teenagers. The paper warned of the potential risks associated with teenag-ers making decisions of this magnitude, and advised ways to ensure these deci-sions are made with maturity and safety in mind.

The second, released in April 2005, warned consum-ers of the dangers associated with plastic surgery tourism. The paper outlined the risks, and ways to ensure patient safety, if choosing cross-border surgical procedures.

which unpigmented blotches appear on the skin. Vitiligo is generally treated with medications, although some severe cases are treated with bleaching (the treatment Jackson claims to have undergone).

There are currently no 12-step programs to deal with BDD and plastic surgery addiction. Today, body dysmorphic disorder is treated with high-dose selective serotonin reuptake inhibitors (SSRIs) or antidepressants such as Prozac. Talk therapy or psychotherapy has proven successful as well to treat this addiction.

The Rise of Lipotourism

Lipotourism, vacation makeovers, medical tourism, "sun 'n' scalpel" tours. These concepts didn't exist before 1997. But since then, and the exponential growth of the cosmetic surgery industry, overseas cosmetic surgery has become one of the most talked-about issues relating to the field. Revered by consumers for its lower prices and the appealing combination of holidays and aesthetic rejuvenation, medical tourism is the bane of North American plastic surgeons' existence. So much so that in the spring of 2005, the American Society of Plastic Surgeons released a briefing paper warning consumers about the potential hazards of cross-border surgery.

Kathleen Jackson didn't heed any of these warnings as she started thinking about plastic surgery. With her 50th birthday on the way, she visited a surgeon from her hometown of Rockville, Maryland, where a chin lift, upper neck liposuction, and eyelid surgery would cost around $10,000. After doing more in-depth research, she discovered Surgeon & Safari, a plastic-surgery resort in Johannesburg, South Africa. The company manages a database of local plastic surgeons, cosmetic dentists, and LASIK eye surgeons with whom prospective patients communicate via e-mail and phone before arriving. Surgeon & Safari is known for their high-class level of service, and once patients arrive, they are treated to chauffeurs, private nurses, and personal chefs. Kathleen was picked up at the airport in a Mercedes and taken to a guesthouse in a Cape Town suburb. It was surrounded by gardens and included the services of a cook/housekeeper. Following a meeting with the doctor, Kathleen spent several hours in surgery (which cost her only $4,000). She had several days of recovery in a private hospital room before returning to her guesthouse, where a nurse tended to her bandages, checked in on her daily, and drove her to appointments. Virtually no plastic surgery patient in North America receives treatment like this.

Run by Lorraine Melvill, Surgeon & Safari is only one of several medical tourism destinations in South Africa. The country is rapidly becoming a top destination for plastic surgery, thanks in part to its weakening currency. "The lower the [value of the] rand falls, the more advantageous it is for people to come," says Gavin Morrison, a former president of the Association of Plastic and Reconstructive Surgeons of Southern

Africa. Melvill says foreign clientele is now reaching 40 to 50 percent of the patients she treats at Surgeon & Safari. Following the trend, similar facilities have been popping up all over the world in such places as Mexico, Thailand, Russia, and Costa Rica. Consumers like Kathleen Jackson are lured by cut-rate prices and a chance to see the world, even if it is through their bandages. Understandably, North American doctors are more than leery about this trend. While South Africa is known worldwide for its excellent medical practices and Surgeon & Safari is one of the best medical tourism companies in the world, other facilities are not as reputable.

It is virtually impossible to be sure about a facility's cleanliness, the surgeon's and anesthetist's skill level or credentials, and the standards of their equipment before arriving at one of these foreign operations. There is usually little to no follow-up with the surgeon, as patients usually fly home before their stitches are removed. For most patients, low prices outweigh these safety concerns. Cheaper labor costs overseas plus a positive exchange rate can mean prices are one-third to one-half of what patients would pay at home. A patient who received a quote for an $8,875 facelift in New York, for example, could have a facelift and a neck lift at Bangkok's Bumrungrad Hospital for just $2,820 (plus airfare).

But this is the bright side of a complicated, and sometimes ugly, phenomenon. One clinic in particular has garnered some especially bad press. Centro de Ginecologia y Obstetricia in Nuevo Laredo, Mexico, lies just across the border from San Antonio, Texas. Lured by the promises of television ads featuring a man who identifies himself as "Dr. Dave," hundreds of women have flocked to this clinic for surgeries at about a third of what they would cost in Texas.

San Antonio's *Express-News*, a local newspaper, ran an in-depth two-month investigation into the clinic in June 2005. The incredible results of their research and reporting were then released on the Associated Press syndicate. The original story followed Lisa, a 51-year-old mother of three. The woman, only identified by her first name, allowed a reporter to observe her surgery and granted hours of interviews. Lisa felt that premature wrinkles would mean men wouldn't be attracted to her, so she decided to have a full-body makeover including a facelift, breast augmentation, tummy tuck, and more. A local surgeon estimated the cost at around $20,000— far beyond Lisa's modest budget. She had almost given up hope when she saw a man calling himself Dr. Dave in a television advertisement for plastic surgery in Mexico.

Lisa thought David Hernandez, co-owner of Centro de Ginecologia y Obstetricia, looked trustworthy. He calls himself Dr. Dave, but he's not a doctor. Rather, he is a businessman and marketing professional handling advertising and scheduling surgeries from an office in San Antonio. According to his advertisements, he has been sending American patients to his Nuevo Laredo clinic for 25 years. Dr. Dave's price for Lisa's procedures was only $8,000. She was persauded.

The *Express-News* sent reporters across the Rio Grande to follow Lisa, who was driven by Hernandez in his Chrysler. The reporters wrote about the two-story cinderblock clinic, Lisa's bare room, and the ants in her bathroom sink.

She met her surgeon, Dr. Jose Luis Villarreal Arroyo, an hour before her surgery. He examined her breasts and decided that she would need larger implants to occupy all the space her loose skin had left. "You're going to have some hooters," Hernandez laughed.

Before surgery, a Spanish-speaking nurse began to prep Lisa by shaving her pubic hair. The *Express-News* reporter translated as Lisa asked why she was being shaved. The nurse told Lisa she was preparing her for liposuction. "No, no liposuction, no liposuction," Lisa said. "*Ay, perdon,*" was the nurse's reply. Lisa asked Hernandez about the incident later on, but he brushed it off, calling it a "miscommunication."

Apparently the nurse was supposed to go to the room next door.

As Villarreal cut through her scalp, peeling back the flesh from her face, a fly buzzed just over her head. The surgeon and surgical nurse batted at the insect and then asked another nurse to kill it. She chased the fly with a spray bottle for a little while, but wasn't able to find or kill the creature.

Lisa's first surgery took five hours, resulting in a facelift, arm lift, breast implants, and eye surgery. The first night after her surgery, blood soaked her pillow and sheets. But Lisa returned for a second round of surgery, resulting in eight procedures in two weeks. As a result of her 10 hours of surgery, Lisa was covered in scars measuring about 8 feet (2.4 m) in total. Photographs show a deep, purple-red gash circling her midriff.

That scar, the result of her tummy tuck, didn't heal properly and it leaked so much fluid that it seeped through the bandages and soaked her pants. She became depressed, and began to get angry with Hernandez and his clinic.

Despite her anger, she went back to Hernandez when the scarring and leaking wounds didn't improve. He sent her back to the clinic in Mexico, where she was given another, stronger prescription for antibiotics. The visit and her growing panic led her to a San Antonio emergency room. There, an American doctor assured her that most of the healing was coming along, but the oozing tummy-tuck wound was problematic. He gave her yet another prescription, saying that the antibiotics given to her in Mexico were supposed to be injected intravenously, and were the wrong kind. Weeks later, Lisa told the newspaper the wound had healed and her recovery scare was over.

This was not the first time Centro de Ginecologia y Obstetricia and Dr. Dave had been under the media microscope. *People* magazine also ran an exposé of the facility in June 2005, running checks on the clinic's certification and licenses. While Centro's doctors are board-certified specialists, according to *People* magazine inspectors found several problems with the facility itself: inadequate barriers between surgical and non-surgical areas, improperly calibrated anesthesia equipment, no backup power generators, and expired vaccines.

Following the story's release, other patients from the Centro contacted *Express-News* with more horror stories. One woman went to the clinic for a tummy tuck, but her sutures wouldn't heal. She returned to the clinic, but Dr. Dave asked her to sign a release form that was written in Spanish. She refused to sign, and he refused to treat her. She eventually went to an emergency room in San Antonio, but is left with what she describes as a "fist-sized" depression of scar tissue on her lower abdomen. Stories surfaced about two other women who died from gangrenous infections after surgeries at a different clinic in Matamoros, Mexico, across the border from Brownsville, Texas. In one of the cases, the woman's skin peeled off when emergency room doctors lifted her from one bed to another.

Because of inadequate record keeping, oversight, and a system that's hostile to lawsuits, the number of injuries or deaths occurring in Mexican clinics is unknown. But U.S. doctors near the border are very aware of the problem. So many patients have required reconstruction that some Texas surgeons have begun to specialize in "secondary repair" to undo damage done during these Mexican procedures. Other surgeons refuse to take cases like this because of liability issues. In some cases, patients face very expensive repair surgeries when they return from Mexican clinics, suddenly making the initial bargain price a great deal steeper.

CHAPTER 3

Case Studies

Often the most high-profile patients of plastic surgery are also the most hush-hush. One California-based surgeon asserts that there is twice as much surgery in Hollywood than what gets reported or admitted. Plastic surgery fanatic Joan Rivers, who goes to see her plastic surgeon for "tune-ups" every six months, was quoted as saying, "Every woman on television over the age of 25 has had something done." Many of these stars aren't confirming that assumption, though. So, in this fractured and cloak-and-dagger industry, it's every surgeon for him or herself, with sometimes disastrous results. Some mistakes are just that: tragic accidents. Others are the result of careless and sometimes cruel treatment that flies in the face of this so-called caring profession. But doctors are not always to blame for plastic surgery nightmares. Some patients don't know when to stop, and their vanity is the cause of their own and sometimes others' demise.

BOTCHED SURGERIES

Olivia Goldsmith and the Manhattan Clinic Deaths

A successful author and public figure, Olivia Goldsmith's death in 2004 proved to be one of the most ironic of plastic surgery's casualties. She was born and raised in Dumont, New Jersey, with the name Randy Goldfield. After graduating from New York University, she met and married a New York businessman named John T. Reid. She began a career as a management consultant at Booz Allen Hamilton, where she rose up the ladder to become the first female partner. She married Reid in 1976; they were married for six years and in divorce court for another seven. The nasty split resulted in her ex-husband keeping most of the spoils including a house, a Manhattan apartment, and a Jaguar car. Olivia received a cash settlement of $300,000.

She moved to London, England, changed her name to Justine Rendal, and started writing fiction. Written under the pseudonym Olivia Goldsmith, *The First Wives Club* was her first novel, a comic satire about three women seeking revenge after their rich ex-husbands leave them for younger partners. It sold millions of copies and became a hit film in 1996 starring Goldie Hawn, Diane Keaton, and Bette Midler. Hawn's character is a plastic surgery fanatic whose lips are so puffed up with collagen, she barely looks human. It was never clear whether *The First Wives Club* was autobiographical, but her message and indignation was apparent: "It's not right," she told the Associated Press in 1996. "You choose a woman who bears your young and then you discard her for a younger, taller, thinner, blonder model."

"We are expected to have jobs now," she said. "We are expected to raise the family. We're responsible for the home, and we have to have thin thighs. Nobody can do it."

Olivia Goldsmith went on to write nine more novels, all shrewd commentaries on society's expectations of women. Plastic surgery is a recurring motif in her writing. No one was better at reinventing herself than Olivia. She rarely kept people in her life for more than a few years and was estranged from her family. She would end longstanding professional and personal relationships suddenly and apparently without reason. She was known for changing her appearance with various colorful wigs and through the plastic surgery she most vocally satirized. She'd had several procedures in the past, including a chin tuck in 1995 to remove fullness around her face.

On January 7, 2004, she went to the Manhattan Eye, Ear, and Throat Hospital in New York City for another chin tuck. Sources say she had just recovered from the flu and had recently undergone gallbladder surgery, but seemed in good health when she entered. Appearances can be deceiving, and the charismatic author lapsed into a coma before the procedure even started. She had opted for general anesthesia, and as her surgeon injected the anesthetic into her neck things went horribly wrong. Olivia went into convulsions and within four minutes, she was comatose. No one at the clinic was able to revive her and she was transferred to Lenox Hill Hospital. Friends and colleagues kept watch by her bedside, hoping she would regain consciousness. The decision about removing her from life support apparently rested with Nan Robinson, her assistant. But on January 15, eight days after she entered the hospital, Olivia Goldsmith died.

A month later Susan Malitz, the 54-year-old wife of a highly respected urologist, died at the same clinic. She too died from complications related to anesthesia. The Manhattan Eye, Ear, and Throat Hospital had enjoyed almost 25 years of spotless reputation, with several celebrity-level plastic surgeons working under its roof. On May 14, 2004, the state of New York fined Manhattan Eye, Ear, and Throat Hospital $20,000 for "egregious violations."

Dying to be thin: Killer Liposuction

At age 47, Judy Fernandez didn't like what she saw in the mirror. She had gained 30 pounds since meeting her husband Ruben, and wasn't happy with the wrinkles she had developed. She'd had her breasts enhanced several years before, and decided to try plastic surgery again.

Judy thoroughly interviewed potential physicians in the Orange County area, researched news stories, and even consulted the California state medical board in hopes of finding a surgeon with a clean track record. The doctor she chose, Dr. William Earle Matory Jr., had been educated and trained at Yale and Harvard. He was also board-certified. What Judy didn't, and couldn't, know was that Matory had also been sued for malpractice four times and had settled once for $32,500.

On March 17, 1997, she entered Matory's New You Plastic Surgery Medical Group in Irvine, California, for liposuction of her thighs, hips, stomach, and buttocks, a facelift, a brow lift, and laser resurfacing. Twelve hours later, she was dead. Her body had been flushed with 5.1 gallons (19 liters) of fluid. It had diluted her blood so extensively, the coroner decided she had bled to death. Her husband was unfortunately privy to the horrific effects of Judy's fatal operation. When he was told that his wife was to be rushed to the hospital, he forced his way into the operating theatre to find her swollen and bleeding.

Judy Fernandez's case went in front of the Medical Board almost immediately and Ruben became incredibly vocal about the negligent death of his beloved wife. He has been interviewed by regional and national newspapers and magazines bringing an issue greater than Judy's death into the public eye. After a 26-day trial, both Matory and anesthesiologist Robert Hoo were charged with gross negligence by the Medical Board of California and stripped of their licenses. Judy Fernandez's death, and others in California, prompted the board to form a special committee to study cosmetic surgery. The debate went national, and Ruben discovered something that may have saved his wife. The National Practitioner Data Bank is a federal government-managed resource of physician information that is off-limits to patients like Judy Fernandez. Today it would reveal Matory's 22 malpractice suits and more than $1 million in settlement pay-outs, even though his license was revoked in December of 1997. Ruben Fernandez testified in front of Congress, pleading with them to open the database to the public, to no avail.

An Associated Press review of the public version of the data bank, which does not reveal doctors' names, found that nearly 500 doctors and dentists across the U.S. have been slapped with at least 10 disciplinary actions and malpractice payments each over the past decade.

RECKLESS PLASTIC SURGEONS

Dr. Death

The story of Judy Fernandez and Earle Matory was only one of the tragedies that opened the California state medical board's inquest. Dr. Patrick Chavis represented another even deadlier side of the problem: uncertified doctors performing unregulated and in some cases reckless plastic surgery.

Patrick Chavis was exalted by national government and media as the poster-boy for affirmative action. In an historic and highly publicized upset, the African-American obstetrician-gynecologist had taken white medical school applicant Allan Bakke's spot as a medical student at University of California, Davis in 1973. UC Davis had begun a special race-based program of admissions that ensured a certain number of spots for minority applicants. Bakke's marks and test scores were better than Chavis's (Bakke scored in the 90th percentile for both the MCAT exam and his college grades), but Chavis got into Davis and Bakke did not. Chavis successfully completed medical school and graduated as an obstetrician/gynecologist (OB/GYN).

The media and politicians loved the story, and he was practically exalted in the *Los Angeles Times*. He was featured in the award-winning documentary *Eyes on the Prize*. Senator Edward Kennedy cited Chavis as an example in April 1996 during a debate over Proposition 209, which proposed the elimination of racial preference.

Like so many other cases of plastic surgeons gone wrong, Chavis's life looked wonderful from the outside. His success had made him a hero in the tough, gang-riddled suburb of Compton. He still lived there, but instead of poverty, he lived in luxury with a large house and fancy cars.

In June 1995, Chavis made the cover of *The New York Times Magazine*, which showed him posed dramatically under surgical lamps holding a newborn baby. The article, written by Nicholas Lemann, presented the doctor as a consummate physician implying that patients couldn't do better than Dr. Patrick Chavis. Interestingly, the story is now regarded as one of the more important pieces of scholarship and debate on the affirmative action issue. Once again, Patrick Chavis was not being evaluated from a medical perspective, but from a political one.

A close look at his real professional reputation would eventually put the politicians and pundits on their heels. On June 19, 1997, Patrick Chavis's license was revoked indefinitely by the California Medical Board. The ruling officially stated that Chavis was unfit to "perform some of the basic duties required of a physician" and allowing him to continue to practice medicine would "endanger the public health, safety and welfare."

Chavis was charged with gross negligence of three of his patients. The first was Yolanda Mukhalian who went into surgery on May 11, 1996, for what she thought would be liposuction of her abdomen. Either through a miscommunication or his own so-called professional judgment, Chavis also sucked fat out of her buttocks, hips, and thighs. The problems began right after surgery. Yolanda's heart was pounding from distress, and fluid and blood began seeping from her incisions and down her legs. Instead of taking her to a hospital, Chavis took her back to his house, where he left her for more than 40 hours. Chavis ignored her frantic phone calls, and she lost 70 percent of her blood. She was lucky to be alive.

On June 21, 1996, Chavis performed liposuction on Valerie Lawrence. Valerie lost an abnormal amount of blood and lost consciousness from massive internal bleeding several hours after being released from surgery. She admitted herself to the hospital in distress, but Chavis discharged her without removing her Foley catheter and IV tubes. Again, Chavis took this patient to his home. The next day, he left her in the care of his 18-year-old niece and went to work.

Tammaria Cotton was a 43-year-old grandmother, who went in for liposuction on June 22, 1996. Her husband Jimmy was with her in the operating room and watched as Chavis and his nurse/girlfriend Carlitha M. Allen administered the anesthetic. Tammaria was in pain and even had trouble breathing during the procedure, but her complaints were ignored and even mocked by Dr. Chavis, who had other things including Valerie Lawrence on his mind. According to an interview by Kenneth Lloyd Billingsley for *Front Page Magazine*, Jimmy Cotton noticed a severe drop in his wife's blood pressure and was horrified by clear, red fluid he saw collecting on the operating room floor. After the surgery, Chavis left the clinic. There were no other support staff or vehicles at the clinic except Carlitha Allen who did very little to help as Tammaria Cotton slowly died of severe abdominal hemorrhage.

Eventually Allen called 911, and when the paramedics arrived, Tammaria's pulse was so faint they thought she was already dead. She was pronounced dead later that evening at St. Francis Hospital.

For a year after Tammaria Cotton's death, Patrick Chavis continue to practice his barbaric form of medicine before the medical board put him under review and stripped him of his license. The investigation revealed an horrific history of almost inhuman disregard for patient suffering. One such example has been written about across the country. Staff from a medical office next door to Chavis's clinic recorded four audio tapes of screaming by patients in the doctor's care. The tapes also feature Chavis's voice saying, "Don't talk to the doctor while he is working" and "Liar, liar, pants on fire." In one case a patient could be heard screaming "stop!" A former colleague told medical investigators that Chavis was "aggressive … careless" and showed "poor impulse control and sensitivity to patients' pain."

Chavis was trained as an obstetrician/gynecologist, but had been performing uncertified liposuction since 1995. His training in liposuction consisted of a four-day course at the Liposuction Institute of Beverly Hills. The second part of the training would have involved 20 liposuction surgeries on his own patients at the Institute's surgery center with an Institute doctor assisting and supervising. But Chavis did not do this. Instead, he began a clandestine after-hours liposuction practice out of an unused surgical suite undergoing renovations.

Chavis's partner was his nurse and girl-friend Carlitha Allen. The California Medical Board revoked her license in 1999 citing gross negligence, incompetence while performing liposuction, and practicing medicine without a license.

After Chavis's medical review, the shocking story was slow to hit the media. Journalist and scholar William McGowan noted that the *Los Angeles Times*, which had lauded Chavis years before for his successes, took more than two months of reporting to identify him as the same Patrick Chavis of affirmative action fame. It seemed all the former Patrick Chavis supporters had disappeared. Shockingly, Chavis himself took the opportunity to cry racism. "I need your help," a self-produced leaflet read. "I have become a political victim of the system and especially the Medical Board of California."

In a striking twist of fate, Chavis was murdered on July 23, 2002, in Hawthorne, California, an economically depressed neighborhood on the southern edge of Los Angeles. He was shot by three men holding up a convenience store. He was buying ice cream.

MD: Mass Destruction

From the outside, Anthony Pignataro had become the respected and successful surgeon his father was. He had all the trappings of success, from a flashy car to private school education for his two children. But, beneath the exterior, Pignataro was neither a healer nor an altruist.

He began losing his hair at the age of 23, and in the early 1990s, Pignataro invented a hairpiece that bolted onto four titanium snaps imbedded into the scalp. He was his own first patient (his father did the implantation of the snaps), and the hairpieces received brief media attention on *The Maury Povich Show*, *Hard Copy*, and elsewhere. Throughout his medical training he was known for alienating his colleagues and he performed poorly during two

failed residencies. Eventually, he set up an uncertified plastic surgery clinic in the basement
of his West Seneca, New York, office.

His professional life had problems right
from the beginning. Mistakes during nose surgery left one patient with brain damage. Two
tummy tuck operations resulted in excessive
bleeding, and there were at least half a dozen
other surgical errors on his record. All of these
mistakes were kept out of the limelight, but following the death of 26-year-old Sarah Smith,
Pignataro's career would take a sharp turn for
the worst. Undergoing a simple breast augmentation, Sarah Smith's heart stopped during
surgery. She became comatose and died several
days later. According to a medical board review,
she didn't have a chance. Her surgery was attended by a nurse and a high school student
working as the office help, and the board determined that there was insufficient anesthesia
support. The case went to criminal court, and
Pignataro pleaded guilty to a charge of crimi-

nally negligent homicide. He was sentenced to six months in prison, and his medical license was revoked.

Pignataro's wife Deborah had publicly supported her husband throughout his trial and conviction. But, after his return from prison, problems with his marriage escalated and he moved out of their home. He had a girlfriend, with whom he lived briefly. However, when he moved back home with Deborah in 1999, it seemed the couple had reconciled. It wasn't so. A short while after his return, Deborah began suffering mysterious symptoms. She was in pain and vomiting. Confused and ill, she went into the hospital on July 21, 1999, where doctors determined she had an inflamed pancreas. She was released, but her symptoms got much worse soon after. She was disoriented and had lost feeling in her limbs. The vomiting continued and the pain became extreme. Two weeks later, she was back in hospital with a shocking new diagnosis. She had been poisoned.

Her husband had been feeding her arsenic, commonly found in ant poison, since he moved back home. Anthony Pignataro pleaded guilty to attempted first-degree assault. He was sentenced to 5 to 15 years in a federal prison. When his wife was admitted to the hospital the first time, Pignataro was adamant the doctors should operate. Medical experts at the subsequent trial said Deborah probably would not have survived a major surgery such as the one Pignataro advocated. The court's prosecutors suggested that a so-called accidental death in the operating room would have vindicated Pignataro from the shame of Sarah Smith's death.

Several years after his conviction, true crime author Ann Rule discovered the Pignataro case and included it in her book *Last Dance, Last Chance*. While researching the story, she uncovered Pignataro's addiction to heroin, which began in prison. According to Rule, Pignataro's plot to kill Deborah had nothing to do with clearing his name. Rather, the doctor had tried to hire someone to kill his wife. When no one would take him up on the offer, the socio-pathic doctor decided to do it himself.

While researching the story, Rule came across a manuscript that had been sent to her in 1997. *M.D.: Mass Destruction* was the story of a doctor whose career is unfairly destroyed by medical licensing boards. When the badly writ-ten manuscript arrived on her desk in 1997, she ignored it, but after Pignataro's conviction, it became more interesting. *M.D.: Mass Destruc-tion* was written by none other than Anthony Pignataro.

PLASTOHOLICS ANONYMOUS

Cindy Jackson: Living Barbie

Cindy Jackson grew up in an Ohio farming community, the daughter of a farmer-turned-inventor and a coal-miner. She describes a childhood characterized by feelings of isolation and never fitting in. When she was six years old,

CINDY JACKSON'S WISH LIST

- Larger, less tired-looking eyes
- A small feminine nose
- High cheekbones
- Fuller, better-shaped lips
- Perfect white teeth
- A smaller, more delicate jaw and chin
- To have just the one chin
- To eradicate premature facial wrinkles and acne scarring
- A flawless, unlined complexion
- A defined waistline and flat stomach
- To lose [her] love handles, saddlebags, and cellulite
- Thinner thighs and slimmer knees
- To get rid of flab left over from being 50 lb overweight
- Not to have to wear a lifetime of hardship etched on [her] face

Source: cindyjackson.com

her parents bought her a Barbie doll. Cindy dreamed of living a happy and glamorous life, just like Barbie. After high school, she attended art college and trained to be a photographer. She worked for a year and a half at menial gas station and factory jobs in order to afford a plane ticket to London, England, and a way out of her drab existence. In England, she continued her art studies and got involved in the punk rock scene. For 10 years, she was in one punk rock band or another, beginning as a backup singer and eventually fronting her own band.

In 1988, Cindy received a small inheritance. This was the beginning of a complete reinvention, which would change more than just her appearance. She put together a wish list based on principles of beauty she learned as an art student and what she refers to as "basic laws of human attraction."

Cindy Jackson says she "made a plan" to systematically correct each of her perceived flaws. She boasts that she fixed every one over the course of 9 operations, although the media has often cited almost 50 operations. Three of the surgeries were done in the late 1980s. Two or more of the operations were to correct the results of the early work. She has had eye lifts, nose jobs, cheek implants, chin reduction, jaw reshaping, facelifts, breast implants put in and removed, fat transfers, and liposuction. She has also had a myriad of non-surgical procedures including dermabrasion, chemical peels, lip enhancement, cosmetic dentistry, and semi-permanent makeup. Her list of procedures reads like a plastic surgery reality show, but Cindy is one of a kind. She is in the *Guinness Book of World Records* for her extensive plastic surgery (and incidentally for having spent the most on a cat. Her cat, Cato, is a second generation Bengal cat that cost her £25,000, equivalent to $45,370 today).

The most interesting part of Cindy Jackson's story isn't that she had the surgery but that she became a celebrity because of it. Now known as "The Living Barbie Doll," Jackson has enjoyed incredible media attention and is paid handsomely for public appearances. She has been photographed with stars such as Michael Jackson and Ivana Trump. She has an exclusive modeling contract and has written a bestselling autobiography, *Living Doll.*

Another woman famous for nothing but her plastic surgery is known as The Cat Lady. The former wife of rich and powerful heir apparent Alec Wildenstein, Jocelyne Wildenstein has purposely transformed her features to resemble a feline. The Wildenstein family was known as secretive, rich, and one of the most powerful art collectors in the world. Their wealth is estimated at $5 billion.

The family's privacy was shattered when Swiss-born Jocelyne returned from vacation to find her husband in a compromising position with a teenage model. The tabloids salivated over the acrimonious divorce. Despite revelations that the couple spent a million dollars a month to sustain their lifestyle and paid no taxes, Jocelyne herself received much of the coverage. To keep herself looking young, and supposedly to appeal to her husband's love of wild cats, she gradually transformed her facial features into that of a feline. Her surgery is so extensive and bizarre, she no longer looks human.

Looks Aren't Everything

Obsession with looking good can be taken too far, as it was in the case of relatively little-known comedian Margaret Trigg. Trigg died in 2003 of unknown causes according to her obituary. But, friends and colleagues knew the real story. In a heartfelt and revealing feature in *New York Magazine*, writer Isadora Fox uncovered the sad reality of a woman's struggle for fame in an industry that demands perfection. Born a rancher's daughter in Bastrop, Texas (population: 6,200), Margaret Trigg was known for her flamboyance, her beauty, and a killer sense of humor. She moved to New York City in 1989 where she found work in a comedy series called "No Shame" performed in a small Soho theater. Her routines were sharp and caustically funny, and she had the talent of transforming herself into a different person while onstage, but she had bigger plans for herself. She wanted to be a star. In order to fit into the impossibly thin mold of a Hollywood starlet, she began abusing laxatives to lose weight quickly. In the beginning, the plan seemed to work. She was signed to the Gersh Agency, a talent agency specializing in comedians. Gersh got her a small role as a prostitute on *Homicide: Life on the Street*, which led to a leading role in an obscure series called *Aliens in the Family*. But, the show was canceled after only a few episodes.

Aliens in the Family had earned her around $120,000, and she used this money to alter her appearance, over and over again. She began with another nose job (she had her first while in high school). Then there was an eye lift, then a brow lift, and then liposuction on her hips and thighs. She had three nose jobs before her surgeon refused to operate on it anymore. She had several more eye lifts. Friends began noticing scarring from too many eye surgeries that Margaret tried to cover up with excessive makeup. In fact, many photographs from the time reveal a makeup-covered face that is many shades lighter than her tanned body. But, she still wasn't satisfied. According to Fox's article, she took a copy of one of her actor's headshots and drew various "improvements" on her nose and chin. Fox writes that the photograph was covered in notes, some as specific as "Eyebrows a few millimeters too arched." She had notebooks filled with drawings and notes as well that read: "I don't want a deep or hollow eye crease. I hate this about upper-lid jobs."

No matter how many surgeries she had, her dream of acting onscreen was over. She got a job reading Tarot cards in a strip club to pay the bills. She kept producing her comedy routines, working at the clubs, and starving herself. Her once-endearing, wacky personality became harsh and strident, and she alienated many of her friends. She was fired from the Gersh agency and went through several shady talent agents, some of whom wanted sexual favors in return for representation. Close friends say she began lying about projects so people would think she was still working.

By April 2002, Margaret's sickness was escalating dangerously. She returned home to Texas to recover from a sleeping pill and Xanax addiction. While in Texas, she was diagnosed with bipolar disorder (manic depression). A psychiatrist in New York would later tell her she had borderline personality disorder. By mid-2002, she was taking several antidepressants, plus antipsychotics and lithium to treat the bipolar disorder. But a few weeks later, she ended up in the psychiatric ward of Bellevue Hospital for a short while. The laxative abuse had damaged her rectum so badly, she was unable to control her bowels. She refused to stick with any of the treatment plans prescribed by the doctors, and her mental state deteriorated. She began talking about suicide. In October 2003, she was readmitted to Bellevue and began therapy. On November 16, her friend Danielle Fenton came to visit. Margaret seemed in good spirits, eating the treats Danielle had brought, wearing colorful pajamas and full makeup. But, later that day, Margaret Trigg was found dead in her hospital bed. Autopsy reports label her cause of death as a heart attack resulting from prolonged amphetamine abuse. The woman who made people laugh had died tragically, wasting her talent and her life in pursuit of an unattainable ideal.

COSMETIC CRIMES

When Beauty Turns Ugly

No matter what she did, Theresa Ramirez hated her breasts. She'd had a mastectomy following a breast cancer diagnosis. She opted for implants as part of her reconstruction, but she was unhappy with them, saying they weren't even. So, she went in for more surgery. Over the course of 8 years, she had 13 breast reconstruction surgeries. After her 13th surgery, she was sure that her implants were leaking, despite her doctor's assurances to the contrary. In fact, nothing the doctors said would convince her that her breasts looked normal. On July 3, 1997, Theresa went to Dr. Michael Tavis's plastic surgery clinic with a gun. She shot and killed him. Later, she attempted suicide and failed. She was arrested and put in jail. In March 1998, Theresa was still detained awaiting trial. Wrapping a sheet from her bedding around her neck, she tried to hang herself from a shower head in the Sonoma County jail's infirmary area. Her second suicide attempt also failed. Theresa went to trial for the first-degree murder of Tavis in 1999. Her lawyers tried to convince the jury that she suffered from body dysmorphic disorder, and the severe mental illness had driven her to violence. The defense failed and she was convicted and sentenced to life in prison.

In Bellevue, Washington, Beryl Challis was horrified by the results of her facelift. Despite almost constant reassurance from her husband and friends, she was devastated. One April morning, she went back to see her surgeon, Dr. Selwyn Cohen, saying she was in pain. He prescribed some painkillers and she left the office. Later that evening, after the clinic had closed, Beryl returned. She knocked on the door and asked him to let her in. She pulled out a .38 caliber handgun and shot Dr. Cohen. Then she drove home and ended her own life. Plastic surgeons have been the targets of criticism from members of society as well as from within the medical profession. Disregarded as an unnecessary practice catering to the vain and the rich, doctors in this field constantly fight for respect and in some cases for their lives.

The 1993 death of one Chicago-area surgeon was linked to a far more insidious and political rationale than the cases of Theresa Ramirez and Beryl Challis. Jonathan Preston Haynes was 34 years old. He had worked for the U.S. Bureau of Alcohol, Tobacco, and Firearms for a couple of years, and he was a neo-Nazi. Haynes was a member of the National Alliance, a group organized by William Pierce, a former physics professor and a member of the American Nazi Party. The National Alliance is one of the largest Nazi organizations in the United States. In August 1993, Haynes flipped through the *Yellow Pages* phone book. Dr. Martin Sullivan had one of the largest ads in the book so Haynes called the office and made an appointment under a false name. On August 6, Haynes went to Sullivan's office and when he was ushered into the examining room, he pulled out a gun and shot the doctor.

A few days later he confessed to police, telling them he shot Sullivan at close range to ensure that he had killed the right man. It was revealed that Haynes had also murdered Frank Ringi, a San Francisco hairdresser, and had been stalking Lake Forest executive Charles Stroupe, the president of the largest manufacturer of blue-tinted contact lenses. He had kept a diary of his murders and had even recorded a cassette tape with a confession and his rationale behind the murders. He said that he intended to send the tape to cosmetic industry executives, warning them to stop "diluting Aryan beauty." During the trial, much of which was used to determine his psychological fitness, he opted to act as his own counsel. His defense consisted mainly of statements regarding his Aryan philosophy. On April 29, 1994, he was found guilty of murder and a week later was sentenced to death. Dr. Martin Sullivan had been the unfortunate victim of an extreme death plan aimed at people who promoted "fake Aryan beauty" through plastic surgery, bleached-blonde hair, and blue-tinted contact lenses.

Crime Lord Cover-Up

In some cases, criminals become the patients and ultimately the victims of plastic surgery procedures. Mexican drug lord Amado Carrillo Fuentes was known to police as the "Capo without a face." No one knew what the 40-something drug trafficker looked like or his real age for that matter. Officials said he smuggled four times more drugs into the United States than any other trafficker in history and his fortune was estimated at $25 billion. Rumors and conjecture surrounded the crime lord, but chances are he wanted it that way. Carrillo was known for ingenuity, and he'd have to be cagey to dodge Mexican government, the U.S.'s Drug Enforcement Agency (DEA), and various assassins for 20 years.

Carrillo became one of the most powerful drug lords in the world, and one of the first to use Boeing 727s and cargo aircraft to move tons of cocaine from South America to Mexico, where supplies were then shipped and trucked across the U.S. border. He forged relations with the Cali cartel in Columbia, and following a crackdown on the Cali dons in 1995, Carrillo had become the number one force in the American cocaine market. DEA agents believe that in 1997 his organization grossed $4 million to $5 million a day. Carrillo first made headlines in November 1993 when he escaped hit men from a rival drug clan in Mexico City. In January 1996, he was in the news again when he disappeared from his sister's wedding just before law enforcers arrived hoping to catch the drug lord unawares.

Mexican authorities say that he even had the head of the country's anti-drug agency, General Jesus Gutierrez Rebollo, on his payroll until the general's arrest in February 1996.

While the Mexican government had tried to set up sting operations to shut him down, because of corruption on many levels, none of these efforts ever amounted to much. American and Mexican initiatives were often at odds, and the two countries never seemed able to cooperate, allowing Carrillo to operate relatively unhindered. Crime lord or not, even Carrillo bowed to the pressures of youth. Entering his forties, Carrillo went in for a facelift and abdominal liposuction in July 1997. Speculation abounds over the reason for the surgery; some thought it was to combat the effects of aging while others speculated he was changing his appearance for a life underground.

Regardless of the reason, Carrillo entered a Mexico City hospital under the name Antonio Flores Montes. Eight hours later, he was dead.

The cause of death was listed as heart failure, but whether it was due to anesthesia complications or complications due to a cocaine habit remains unknown. In fact, everything about Carrillo's death, including the cause, was debated. Some people even thought his two bodyguards, present during the surgery, administered a fatal overdose of drugs. When Mexican and American officials arrived to identify the body, it was beyond recognition. The tip of his nose was completely gone, and his eyelids were badly bruised and scarred. Incisions for a chin implant had been opened during the autopsy and then re-sutured using white thread. Carrillo's mother, Aurora, identified the body as her son's, but the prevailing thought was that Carrillo had faked his own death.

Despite all the rumor and conspiracy theories, Thomas Constantine, the head of the U.S. Drug Enforcement Agency, confirmed that the body's fingerprints matched those on a border-crossing card from Carrillo's early days in the drug trade. The man who had dodged authorities and assassins in two countries for years had met his end on a plastic surgeon's operating table.

CHAPTER 4

A System Out of Control?

The field of plastic and cosmetic surgery is largely unregulated and in some cases drastically untracked. Most of the certifying bodies and professional associations operate on voluntary memberships, and for consumers it is frighteningly buyer beware, as even certified surgeons aren't necessarily competent. The National Practitioner Data Bank, which houses critical information about malpractice claims against specific physicians in the U.S., is not accessible to the general public. On top of that, many private surgical facilities are not certified and thousands of procedures done in doctor's offices happen literally off the radar of monitoring organizations.

In the United States and Canada, licensure and certification are monitored similarly. A medical license is the minimum standard necessary to practice medicine. It falls under public jurisdiction and is administered at the state or provincial level. Certification, which is distinct from having a medical license, is for specific medical specialties. In the U.S., certification is done by the American Board of Medical Specialties (ABMS), an umbrella organization for 24 approved medical specialties including plastic surgery. The Canadian system is administered by the Royal College of Physicians and Surgeons. Both the ABMS and the Royal College dictate educational, practical, and ethical requirements for a specialist in a specific medical field.

The general requirements for plastic surgery certification are that the doctor's major professional activity is plastic surgery, and that doctor must maintain an ethical and moral standard acceptable to the Board and/or College. Specific requirements include graduation from an accredited medical school and at least five years of postgraduate surgical training.

Most consumer-focused plastic surgery resources advise people to engage a "board-certified" doctor for their procedures. However, "board-certified" doesn't necessarily mean the doctor is a board-certified, trained plastic surgeon. The doctor could be a board-certified gynecologist, as was the case with Dr. Patrick Chavis. Even though he was a specialist, he had absolutely no formal training in surgery, let alone plastic surgery, and had only a four-day course in liposuction to instruct him.

In the U.S., legislation regulating the practice of plastic surgery occurs at a state level. That means every state controls and limits

SUMMARY OF DIFFERENCES IN U.S. STATE LAWS

California law dictates that all non-hospital surgical centers that use sedation or general anesthesia must be accredited by the AAAASF. Florida, Georgia, Pennsylvania, New York, and Texas law reflects the same standard.

Sixteen states, including Alaska, Colorado, Oregon, and Arizona allow dental surgeons to perform plastic surgery. Seventeen states require that plastic surgeons are trained and board certified specifically in plastic surgery. Seventeen others are either in the midst of legislation debate on the issue, or have been targeted by dental surgeons to challenge current legislation.

Source: The Coalition for Safe Plastic Surgery

the practice differently. Only 17 of the 50 states have legislation in place to guarantee that only board-certified MDs with a specialization in plastic surgery are authorized to perform cosmetic procedures. Sixteen states have laws that are so lax, dental surgeons are permitted to perform cosmetic plastic surgery.

In addition to the government and professional certifying boards, plastic surgeons have a bewildering array of professional associations with intimidating and convincing acronyms: ASAPS, CSAPS, AAPS. Most professional associations, such as the American Society of Aesthetic Plastic Surgeons (ASAPS), require that their members be board-certified plastic surgeons. Membership usually has dual purposes, attempting to educate and protect both the public and its members. The trouble is, it is generally not the board-certified surgeons that the public need worry about but rather the uncertified physicians who operate independently of these organizations. And the professional organizations can do little but issue ineffectual press releases warning consumers about the dangers of uncertified physicians. Also, protecting their members sometimes means disregarding serious consumer concerns, as was the case with the silicone-gel breast implant scare. Scientific studies clearly showed no health risks associated with breast implants, but the professional fraternity of plastic surgeons was perceived as the "medical mafia" nonetheless.

Regardless, the surgeon is only half the story. The other part of the equation of patient safety is the surgical facility itself. In the United States, the growth of private outpatient surgical facilities has been dramatic. In 1983, there were 239 freestanding surgical centers performing approximately 377,000 surgical procedures. By 2002, there were 3,493 freestanding centers. There were also at least 15,000 medical practices with in-office surgery suites.

During a 6-month period in 2002, 5 people died and 15 people were seriously harmed during office surgeries in Florida. Since 1997, more than 30 people have died following or during cosmetic surgery in the sunshine state. The problem is not confined to Florida; similar numbers of patients have died in New York, Pennsylvania, and California. Some state legislatures have scrambled to increase the controls and some have even temporarily banned certain procedures, but there are just too many facilities to monitor.

The American Association for Accreditation of Ambulatory Surgery Facilities (AAAASF) was established in 1992 in an attempt to standardize and improve the quality of medical and surgical care in outpatient surgery facilities. Today, only 900 outpatient surgery facilities are accredited by AAAASF compared to the more than 3,000 freestanding facilities and thousands of office-based surgical suites in operation. The AAAASF is a non-profit organization with only six staff members and a volunteer board consisting entirely of doctors. The Canadian Association for Accreditation of Ambulatory Surgical Facilities (CAAASF) is a national organization formed in 1990. It is a voluntary organization of doctors, and all members of the executive board are plastic surgeons. There are only 50 accredited surgical facilities in Canada.

One of the greatest benefits of the United States' private health care system is the comprehensive market research done to maintain a clear picture of the market. In Canada, however, elective surgery such as laser eye surgery, dental surgery, and cosmetic surgery falls into a gray area between the private sector and the public health system. Research shows that private health care spending in Canada is as much as 30 percent of total health care spending, but there is no information available on private facilities and what goes on there.

Each year, questions about private health care are set out in the Health Minister's annual report to Canadian Parliament. Each year, the provinces answer these questions the same way: "Number of private surgical facilities—not available. Total payments to private health care facilities—not available."

Several provinces have done their own ad hoc reporting, but the statistics reveal gross inconsistencies. Wendy Armstrong of the Alberta branch of the Consumers Association of Canada set out to write a report on the growth of private clinics in Alberta in 2002. Her project was supposed to take three months and ended up

taking two years. "Why would nobody col-
lect this data?" she asked. "To the best of my
knowledge, I've done the most comprehensive
research on this." And it was only comprehensive up to a point. The most recent statistics
Armstrong found were from 1999, and the study
itself focused on cataract surgery, not cosmetic,
leaving the picture of private plastic surgery
clinics as muddy as ever.

Advertising and Ethics

Before the 1980s, medical advertising and pro-
motion of doctors' practices was unheard of due
to the American Medical Association's (AMA)
"Principles of Medical Ethics." This banned all
advertising by doctors. Beginning in the mid-
1970s, the Federal Trade Commission (FTC)
got involved, filing a number of health care antitrust cases to enforce free trade in medicine.
In fact, the American Society for Plastic and
Reconstructive Surgery (ASPRS) was accused
of antitrust violations based on its requirement

of board certification for membership, now its single most relevant feature.

In 1975, the Supreme Court ruled that prohibiting professional advertising was an illegal restraint of trade. This fueled the FTC's fire, and it successfully overturned the AMA's position in 1982, for better or for worse. The ruling changed the nature of competition in the medical profession, letting physicians act as salespeople and pitch their services directly to consumers. Soon after, the health care system introduced managed care, and with it came a huge decline in doctor reimbursements from health insurers. The plastic surgery business was put in an interesting situation: insurers were paying less for medically necessary procedures and nothing for purely elective ones.

Since then, physician entrepreneurship has become a reality, and no single group stands to profit more than plastic surgeons. Plastic surgery advertising touts the transformative powers of cosmetic work, promising a new life and a new sense of identity. Common marketing practice uses discounts, contests, and special offers to trigger sales. But when plastic surgery advertising collides with medical ethics and legal liability, some potentially disastrous results ensue.

Indianapolis surgeon Dr. Wally Zollman, for example, was the master of advertising and discount plastic surgery. With a huge surgical center bearing his name, large homes, expensive cars, and a world-renowned art collection, he was doing very well. He was well respected in his field and was a media darling, quoted as an expert in *USA Today* and featured in *Forbes* magazine in a story about his tribal mask collection. Zollman's collection was worth millions, one of the largest of its kind in the country. His surgical center had a 1,600-square-foot (150-sq-m) art gallery that employed a full-time curator.

Zollman entered practice while the ban on medical advertising was still in place, and when the ban was lifted in the early 1980s, he took full advantage. His success came not only from his large-scale advertising campaign, but also his upscale, self-named surgical facility, the Zollman Center for Plastic and Hand Surgery. In many ways, Zollman was ahead of his time. His center was able to provide an extensive array of cosmetic procedures, completely unique in the American Midwest. In the early 1990s, he was profiled by *Indianapolis Monthly* as one of the city's top and more visionary doctors. The article claimed that Zollman predicted the boom in cosmetic surgery, and had essentially captured the market in the area. Zollman advertised discounts and promotions, even offering two-for-one specials on breast implants at one point.

However, his next brush with fame would not prove to be as flattering. In early 1995, 32-year-old Kelly Vaughn went to the Zollman Center for liposuction. At the time, she was working for a local television station and thought her experience would make a good story. A camera crew from the station accompanied Kelly on the morning of her surgery. But everything wasn't as it seemed for the cameras.

Kelly Vaughn went in for a relatively minor liposuction procedure to remove some excess fat from her abdomen. When she walked out of the Zollman Center, however, almost 20 pounds of fat had been removed from her back, buttocks, hips, and thighs. Kelly, an African-American, was horrified at the new size of her rear end. She spoke openly about the experience in the very same magazine that had lauded Zollman's achievements several years before. She told *Indianapolis Monthly* writer Maureen Hayden that the African-American standard of beauty reveres a curvy figure and a round derriere. "Don't touch my butt," she said to Zollman before her surgery. "For a black woman, that's like death."

Even though she was upset with the results, the viewers of Channel 59 didn't know it. After promoting her surgery with Zollman so much, she felt pressured to speak positively in public.

In April of 1996, she received an anonymous letter from a nurse at the Zollman Center. The letter informed her that Zollman didn't perform her liposuction: it was a surgical technician named Rex Haller. The letter went on to say that Haller had been directed by Zollman to do surgeries on other patients as well, without their knowledge. This time, Kelly Vaughn went public. She hired a lawyer and went to several local television stations with the story including WISH Channel 8 and Indy Channel 6.

The exposé brought Zollman's empire and his reputation crashing down. Indy Channel RTV6 ran a report revealing that Zollman had more than 40 lawsuits filed against him, and had settled one case for $575,000. Channel 8 health reporter Debbie Knox found a reprimand from an ethics committee of the American Society of Plastic Surgeons for one of Zollman's large-volume liposuction advertisements. According to Knox, the ASPS had found that the ad, in which he claimed to be able to remove up to 20 pounds of fat, was "false and misleading."

The media exposure led to more and more of Zollman's patients coming forward with complaints, and in 1997 more than 10 malpractice suits were filed against the doctor. According to the 2004 *Indianapolis Monthly* story, one patient claimed that an infection in her breasts caused her incisions to leak a foul-smelling discharge and turned her nipples black with decay.

The scathing exposé also reported that eight physicians had resigned from the Zollman Center between October 1996 and July 1997. At least one of them sued Zollman for yet another example of the doctor's shady business practices. According to Dr. Michael Beckenstein, Zollman told him that the 1995 profit from his practice was $6 million. But, Zollman was losing money, not making it, and filed for Chapter 11 bankruptcy in March 1999. As part of the filing procedure, he was asked to reveal his debts and assets. He offered the debt information freely, but was reticent with his assets. Finally, further investigation by the courts revealed more than

200 art objects stashed in his various homes, including a trunk full of gold pieces. The total value of the art: $3 million.

The case was turned over for criminal investigation and Zollman's medical license was up for review. He appeared before the medical board in April of 2004. And then ... nothing. As of August 2005, the Indiana Medical Licensing Board lists Zollman's license as "Active," and it isn't up for renewal until 2007. Although his record does state that he has had previous disciplinary action, it doesn't go into details. Today, Zollman continues to practice as a plastic surgeon and his three websites promise immediate call-back to prospective clients. He has numerous advertisements on the Internet, and he even hosted a seminar on breast augmentation in July 2005. What is possibly the most disconcerting aspect of this case is that Zollman was a highly trained, board-certified plastic surgeon with a great reputation before his negligence was brought to light.

The Yellow Pages Stand Trial

Michelle Knepper started her search for a board-certified plastic surgeon in the *Yellow Pages*. There she found an ad that appealed to her and a doctor who she thought fit the bill. That doctor was a dermatologist who, while board-certified for dermatology, had no formal training in liposuction, the procedure Michelle was looking for. She called his office, and both the office manager and later the doctor himself confirmed that he was a board-certified plastic surgeon.

Michelle's liposuction did not go well. The doctor removed too much fat from her thighs and buttocks. In places, the over-suctioning was so severe that Michelle's nerves were nearly exposed, causing constant pain. She underwent two corrective procedures, both of which only worsened her condition. Her injuries were believed to be irreparable, and the cost of corrective work sat at $100,000.

In an unprecedented move, Michelle filed

suit not only against the doctor but against the *Yellow Pages* publisher as well. When the dermatologist placed his ad in the *Yellow Pages,* he wanted it placed under "dermatology," but the ad sales representative encouraged him to list it under "plastic surgery," thus contributing to the doctor's fraud. This dermatologist was not an isolated case, either. The *Yellow Pages* frequently encouraged doctors to advertise in areas outside their field of expertise, violating their own code of ethics. The *Yellow Pages'* vice president even testified that the company will knowingly allow any physician to advertise in any medical specialty. The jury found in favor of Michelle Knepper, and the *Yellow Pages* was fined $1.6 million.

CHAPTER 5

A History of the Industry

The beauty business has exploded in the past two decades due in part to plastic surgery, but the quest for beauty is as old as time. Makeup, fashion, diet, and hairstyles have been important to people throughout history and the idea of reconstructing our exteriors has been in practice for centuries. In many cases, it had as much to do with the quest for honor as with the quest for beauty. Since ancient times, the nose was considered to be the location of a man's character or reputation. Amputation of the nose, or rhinokopia, aimed to strip a man of his honor and was a more humiliating punishment than death. Rhinokopia is referred to throughout history all over the world in as disparate places as India, Turkey, China, and Islamic countries. For example, Byzantine Emperor Justinian II Rhinotmetus (685–695 and 705–711) was defeated in battle and his nose amputated, earning him the name Rhinotmetus or The Split-Nosed. An ancient marble statue of Justinian reveals the presence of a forehead scar and the suggested form of a reconstructed nose.

Not surprisingly, rhinoplasty, or reconstruction of the nose, was among the first plastic surgery procedures to be performed. In early Indian Sanskrit texts, possibly written more than 2,600 years ago, there are descriptions of nose, ear, and lip reconstructions using skin flap techniques that are still practiced today.

Wartime Resurgence

Plastic surgery and indeed surgery in general experienced a huge decline in the Middle Ages due to intense religious opposition. In fact in the 1500s, surgeons were relegated to the same guild and status as barbers, hence the term barber surgeons. But the World Wars changed all of that with the sheer scope of human casualty. Plastic surgery came into its own during Word War I due mainly to a man named Sir Harold Delf Gillies. Sir Gillies centralized reconstruction patients who had been injured in the war in Western Europe into one facility. There, he treated more than 5,000 people, all the while training surgeons and making huge innovations in the field. He was also well known for his sense of humor and his tendency to name pedicles (skin flaps used in reconstructive surgery). If they failed, the pedicles would receive a funeral reading: one epitaph was to Horace, "to whom I was so attached." After the World Wars, plastic surgery was finally recognized as a legitimate medical specialty. In the 1950s, the field of plastic surgery began to diverge. Reconstructive plastic surgery benefited from the advent of microsurgery, using microscopes to aid in precise reconstruction. And cosmetic surgery became a branch all of its own.

History of Liposuction

The process of removing excess fat from localized body sites was rife with accidents until the mid-1970s. In 1921, French surgeon Charles Dujarrier attempted to remove fat from a dancer's calves and knees. Dujarrier used a uterine curette (a surgical instrument shaped like a spoon, used to remove tissue from a body cavity) and damaged the dancer's femoral artery. The tragic result of this botched surgery: amputation of one of the dancer's legs. Other attempts resulted in hematomas, swelling due to broken blood vessels, and significant scarring.

This all changed in 1974 when father and son gynecologists Giorgio and Arpad Fischer developed a blunt hollow cannula (a small flexible tube) equipped with suction. Liposuction was born. Calling it liposculpture, the method was published in medical journals in 1976 and saw fewer complications than early curette attempts. Giorgio Fischer still practices liposculpture today in Italy and uses a method where his patients receive the treatment standing up to ensure better aesthetic results.

Yves Illouz, a French plastic surgeon in Paris, was interested in the Fischers' innovation but further developed their "dry method." He favored a "wet technique" in which a solution of saline and hyaluronidase (an enzyme that increases tissue absorption of fluids) was introduced into the fatty tissue before suction. Illouz felt this would facilitate fat removal, while reducing trauma and bleeding.

The first American to visit France and learn the new liposuction technique was California dermatologic surgeon Lawrence Field in 1977. In mid-1982, a group of physicians from different specialties received instruction from Illouz and Dr. Pierre Fournier, a world leader in liposuction and fat transplantation. Then, a task force from the American Society of Plastic and Reconstructive Surgeons visited Europe to investigate this new procedure. Excited by its potential, they attempted to monopolize the field by having the French doctors sign a contract to exclusively teach plastic surgeons. Fournier refused to sign the contract and continued to teach physicians from many different fields. Julius Newman, an otolaryngologist and cosmetic surgeon, and his associate Richard Dolsky, a plastic surgeon, taught the first American course on liposuction in Philadelphia in 1982. The first live surgery workshop was held in Hollywood, California, in June 1983 under the direction of the American Society of Cosmetic Surgeons and the American Society of Liposuction Surgery.

Although the process was innovated by Illouz, dermatologist Dr. Jeffrey Klein is credited with the advent of "tumescent" anesthesia in 1987. Tumescent anesthesia involves the introduction of a dilute solution of lidocaine and epinephrine into the fatty tissues acting as a local anesthetic, reducing bleeding even further. This allowed doctors to perform liposuction over larger body areas without the risks of using a general anesthetic.

Complications of liposuction performed with a pure tumescent technique have been minimal. However, the ideal liposuction patient is healthy, in generally good shape, and only 10 to 20 pounds overweight. It is best performed under local anesthetic in an office-based, outpatient setting. The most significant complications with liposuction have been due to unnecessary general anesthesia for large volume liposuction. Deaths have also been associated with liposuction performed concurrently with tummy tuck operations. Hospital-based liposuction, which usually involves general anesthesia, results in 3.5 times as many malpractice claims as office-based procedures.

Breasts Through the Ages

The history of breast enhancement is as long as it is ridiculous. From stuffing bras to suction-based "growth" machines, a large and perky bosom has long been the aesthetic holy grail. In 1877, Sherwood Ferris of Brooklyn, New York, created pads with a substructure of wire or whalebone, paper-machéd into the desired shape and buttoned into a corset. Marie Tucek of New York City engineered the first push-up bra in 1893. It was made of either sheet metal or cardboard and covered with silk. Film stars of the 1950s were envied for their incredibly perky breasts, enhanced by the bras of the day, and in 1968 the advent of the original Wonderbra brought cleavage to America. The erect-nipple aesthetic has been popular with women since at least the 1960s when Maidenform marketed its "Half-Way" model, "a bra for extroverts." More recently, after a trip to Las Vegas, small-busted friends Julia Cobbs and Lori Barghini invented nipple enhancers, nipple-shaped tips that suction onto the breasts and draw attention to any bust line. The enhancers were featured on a 2001 episode of *Sex and the City*, and a Manhattan boutique sold 800 pairs in one week.

The surgical history of breast augmentation is fraught with more hazard but just as much creativity. Three different means of breast augmentation have been attempted, with varying success, in the modern era of plastic surgery: autogenous tissue, injectable synthetic materials, and implantable prosthetic devices.

The earliest attempt to increase breast size in modern times was the use of autogenous tissue (tissue from the patient's own body) by Dr. Vincenz Czerny in 1895. He transplanted fat from a patient's back to her breast to correct an asymmetry. Other surgeons attempted transplanting fat from the buttocks or abdomen to the breast, but they found that it was quickly reabsorbed by the body, resulting in unsightly lumps and bumps with scars left at both the implant and donor sites. Now the only use of autogenous breast surgeries uses muscle tissue from the abdomen and back to aid in post-mastectomy breast reconstructions.

Dr. Robert Gersuny—an Austrian physician—developed the use of paraffin wax injections for breast augmentation in the 1890s. He was followed by others who injected a variety of other substances including beeswax and vegetable oil. Complications were numerous, lead by a high infection rate, and the procedure was discontinued.

In 1943, the Corning Glass Works company joined with the Dow Chemical Company to form the Dow Corning Corporation, and together they pioneered the development of silicone as an engine lubricant that was resistant to high temperatures. Considered an inert material that could be easily sterilized, Japanese cosmetologists injected the liquid directly into women's breasts. Silicone injections gained an underground popularity in World War II among Japanese prostitutes and in the

TIMELINE OF THE SILICONE-GEL BREAST IMPLANT SCARE

1962	Silicone-gel-filled breast implants first used
1976	Medical Devices Amendments give FDA authority to regulate breast implants
1984	Stern vs. Dow Corning. Plaintiff is awarded over $1.7 million for a claim that ruptured implants caused connective tissue disease
1988	FDA re-classifies silicone implants as a Class III device requiring manufacturers to submit safety information
11/1991	Manufacturers' safety information deemed inadequate by FDA
01/1992	FDA imposes a moratorium on silicone implants
02/1992	First class action suit filed in the wake of FDA moratorium. Eventually 440,000 women join.
04/1992	Silicone implants withdrawn from the market except in limited cases
1994	Mayo clinic study shows health risks aren't likely
1995	Dow Corning files for Chapter 11 bankruptcy
2000	U.S. Department of Health study reveals no connection between breast implants and autoimmune disease
2000	Two saline breast implants approved by FDA
2004	Nationwide debate ensues as FDA approves one silicone breast implant from Inamed
2005	FDA conditionally approves Mentor Corp's silicone breast implant

early 1960s among topless dancers in San Francisco and Las Vegas. By the mid-'60s, reports of serious complications—including chronic inflammation and tumor-like lumps and infections that can necessitate mastectomy, as well as organ damage resulting from migration of the silicone—pushed the method out of mainstream medicine.

The last of the three methods of augmentation, implantable prosthetic devices, have certainly been the most successful. The first prosthetic devices were made of ivory or glass, but these materials were abandoned because of the highly unnatural appearance that they produced. Focus then shifted to spongelike materials, such as Ivalon, which could be fabricated to create a more natural appearance of the breast. However, use of sponge-type implants was eventually abandoned because of the late effects of shrinkage, hardening, and distortion due to scar tissue forming around the device itself.

In 1961, Baylor University surgical student Frank Gerow squeezed a plastic blood bag and remarked how much it felt like a woman's breast. By that time, medical-grade silicone had been developed and was being used to treat skin imperfections. Gerow and his mentor, Thomas Cronin, unveiled the silicone breast implant in 1962.

Silicone breast implants, and indeed breast implants in general, have a checkered history. The evolution of modern silicone-based implants began in 1963, when Cronin and Gerow introduced an implant filled with gel, with both the outer shell and inner gel material composed of silicone. In 1964, global silicone supplier Dow Corning began making and marketing silicone breast implants. The implants only represented about one percent of its business, but that tiny percentage would become the corporation's biggest nightmare. When Dow Corning released its implants, the U.S.'s Food and Drug Administration (FDA) did not regulate medical devices. That authority came in 1976, and that same year the FDA classified silicone implants as a class II device, requiring only general controls and performance standards. That classification changed in 1988 and the new requirements were more demanding. The FDA now demanded that manufacturers submit studies on safety and effectiveness.

In early 1989, an unpublished study about polyurethane foam-covered implants raised the FDA's eyebrows. The product was removed from the market, but only a year later, breast implant safety became a huge public concern. Exposing the horrors of breast implants, *Face to Face with Connie Chung* sparked a nationwide outcry. Women all over the United States came forward with claims of chest pain, numbness, and diagnoses such as chronic fatigue syndrome, fibromyalgia, lupus, and multiple sclerosis. In 1992, silicone implants were pulled from the market, to be used only for breast reconstructions as part of a clinical trial. By 1994, Dow Corning was buried beneath an enormous class-action suit with about 400,000 claimants suing for damages. The company filed for Chapter 11 bankruptcy in 1995 and in 1998 settled for $3.2 billion payable to 170,000 women.

Meanwhile, the medical community scrambled to explain the phenomenon. Studies were conducted in the United States and abroad about the safety of breast implants and their relationship to connective tissue diseases and autoimmune diseases. In 1992 the United Kingdom's (UK) Department of Health released an animal study revealing that silicone did not affect immune responses. It also found no evidence of increased risk of connective tissue disease. A 1997 study conducted by the Independent Review Group in the UK also found no link between breast implants and connective tissue disease. A 2000 study by the U.S. Department of Health and Human Services found no evidence that silicone implants caused autoimmune disease, either. The study reported that the primary safety issues were complications such as rupture and capsular contracture, distortion due to scar tissue forming around the implant. The medical community had proven thousands of women wrong. The result was a kind of underground activism spearheaded by individual, outraged women whose principal forums were their homemade websites. One woman, however, transformed her outrage into a national-scale protest.

Sybil Goldrich was diagnosed with advanced breast cancer more than 20 years ago. She had a double mastectomy at age 44 and then consulted plastic surgeons about silicone-gel implants. Breast implants had been the prevailing method of breast reconstruction since the 1960s, and her doctors assured her the implants would last a lifetime. This was the common belief in the 1980s, and a belief that prevailed until the mid-1990s. But breast implants did not last forever. In fact, in many cases they ruptured or leaked and needed to be removed or replaced. Seventy-four percent of silicone breast implants ruptured within 10 years of insertion. Many women are not even aware that an implant has begun to leak until the removal surgery, as was the case with actress Pamela Anderson.

Some time after her surgery, Sybil Goldrich developed a fever and a rash. Her breast had become grotesquely uneven and misshapen. She went through four sets of implants in an effort to reconstruct her disfigured breasts and she endured fever, rashes, and a buildup of scar tissue that left her in excruciating pain.

In 1984, through with implants, Sybil opted for a "tram flap" breast reconstruction operation in which tissue from the abdominal muscles is used to rebuild the chest wall. A mammogram that same year showed that Sybil had breast cancer in six places. During a hysterectomy in May 1988, the doctors found silicone in her uterus, ovaries, and liver. The silicone from her breast implants had leaked throughout her body. Appalled and enraged, Sybil turned her anger into activism. She wrote an account of the experience in *Ms.* magazine. After the article, she was contacted by hundreds of women who had also suffered after breast-implant surgery. In 1988, she and nurse Kathleen Anneken started Command Trust Network, a national breast implant information clearinghouse. Since the late 1980s, Sybil Goldrich has been one of the most vocal anti-silicone activists in the country. She has been interviewed frequently for national newspapers and even revealed her scarred, disfigured breasts on national television. In 1997, Lifetime television network aired a dramatic made-for-TV movie based on her story, called *Two Small Voices.* The role of Sybil was played by actress Mary McDonnell.

After the silicone ban of the early 1990s, the implant business shifted its focus to saline-filled silicone-barriered implants. Doctors could insert saline implants while deflated through a smaller incision, and in some cases through the belly button. The fact that they are filled with saline (essentially salt water) decreased safety concerns as well. But companies continued to try to clear silicone's name in the area of breast implants. In spring of 2005, after 13 years off the market, the FDA reopened the debate on silicone-gel implants. Two companies, Mentor Corporation and Inamed Corporation, applied for approval on two silicone-gel implants. Women across the country representing both sides of the debate attended the FDA's advisory panel meeting. Those who had experienced no trouble with their implants said women should have the right to choose between saline and the more natural-looking silicone gel. Those who had health problems, leakage, and rupture fought to keep silicone off the market.

Dr. Susan Kolb, a plastic surgeon in Atlanta who specialized in implant removals, was happy with her silicone implants for 10 years and even touted their safety to the media. But then she began having problems with her own implants. In 1995, Kolb felt a burning in her chest and numbness in one arm. "I knew they were leaking; I'd had patients with the same symptoms," she said. She says she suffered fatigue, mental clouding, dizziness, and hair loss, and eventually had her implants removed in 1997. Carolyn Wolf, now 74, had her implants put in more than 30 years ago after a mastectomy. She was problem-free for the first seven years before she discovered blisters on her neck and boil-like growths on her forehead. She was admitted to an intensive care unit due to intense chest pain. After that frightening ordeal, she was plagued by excruciating pain in her left eye. A string of silicone, about an inch (2.5 cm) long, came out of that eye. Then silicone started coming out of her ears. Wolf had her severely ruptured implants removed in 2000, but she still suffers from short-term memory loss that she attributes to the implants. "Please," she told the panel, "do not inflict this on another generation."

After three days of testimony from the public, FDA staff, and the two contending manufacturers, the FDA Advisory Panel issued two decisions. On April 12, the FDA voted to deny Inamed's application in a 5–4 decision. The next day, in a 7–2 vote, the FDA approved Mentor's silicone-gel implant with a set of conditions including a training and certification requirement before surgeons could receive the product. The FDA also required Mentor Corp. to complete a 10-year study and convene with the FDA in 5 years to review the data. Mentor Corp. was also required to establish an independent safety committee and obtain follow-up information on patients that had their implants removed.

Silicone gel-filled breast implants won conditional approval from the FDA to return to the U.S. market after a 13-year ban when health officials backed a version made by Mentor Corp on July 28, 2005.

The Botox® Story

Alastair and Jean Carruthers met in medical school in Vancouver, British Columbia, in the

mid-1970s. Alastair was just finishing his studies to become a dermatologist and Jean an
ophthalmologist. The couple married and had
three sons, meanwhile setting up practices in
the bustling Canadian city. In 1982, Alastair was
invited to do postgraduate study in microsurgery in San Francisco. Jean followed, joining
the Smith Kettle Wells Institute for Visual Sci-
ences to learn about new uses for Botulinum A
Extoxin in the treatment of misaligned eyes. In
1982, Jean brought the toxin back to Canada for
use in a clinical trial involving misaligned and
spasming eyes.

In 1987, one of Jean's patients asked for the
toxin to be injected into her eyebrow. Confused,
Jean said it wasn't necessary because her brow
area wasn't in spasm. "I know it's not in spasm,"
said her patient. "But every time you treat me
there I get this beautiful untroubled expres-
sion." And, quite by accident, Botox® was born.

Jean went home and mentioned the idea
to Alistair over dinner. He was thrilled with

the prospects, but first they'd have to try it on someone. Jean's receptionist Cathy had deep creases in her forehead. She'd seen the stream of patients coming out of Jean's office and offered to be the guinea pig. At first, members of the dermatological surgery community to whom she initially presented the idea thought she was crazy. But massive, widespread acceptance soon followed, and FDA approval came in Canada in 2001 and the United States a year later. Botox® is now widely used to treat wrinkles acutely on the forehead, cheeks, mouth area, and chin. It is also injected into armpits to decrease

BOTULINUM A AND B

Clostridium botulinum is a bacteria that causes botulism. It produces seven different neurotoxins that act as paralyzing agents, called simply Botulinum A, B, C1, D, E, F, and G.

Botulinum A, commonly known as Botox, was approved by the FDA for use in blepharospasm (spasming eyes) and wrinkles.

Botulinum B, known as Mybloc or Neurobloc, is used for cervical dystonia, involuntary movements, spasm, and abnormal posture of the head and neck.

perspiration. The action of the toxin is one of temporary paralysis, lasting about three months. Botox® has been criticized for its overuse, resulting in expressionless faces and, if poorly administered, drooping, uneven eyes.

One of the more recent phenomena is that of the "Botox® party"—doctor-hosted social gatherings where each guest pays for one or more Botox® injections. Touted as the Tupperware party of the new millennium, Botox® parties gained popularity because of the relative ease of the procedure. But the parties have received their share of criticism for trivializing a serious medical procedure that should be administered in a controlled office environment. However, doctors stand to benefit handsomely from the events, often earning several hundred dollars per guest.

CHAPTER 6

The Future

Cosmetic surgery has changed drastically in the past two decades, both as a field of study and an industry. Advancements in technology mean better and safer implantable devices as well as more effective methods that reduce healing time and risk.

As a result of the decade-long silicone-gel breast implant debate, implants now feature stronger barrier shells that are more resistant to rupture and deflation. Implant design has also improved. Some implants feature a textured exterior surface designed to reduce the chance of scar tissue hardening around the implant. Saline-filled implants already feature valves for relatively easy resizing, reducing the need for full-scale corrective surgeries to increase or decrease size. As design and safety improves, breast implants will become more customizable, longer lasting, and safer.

The major recent advances, though, have been in the field of injectable cosmetic treatments. Safe, quick, and requiring little downtime, injectables such as Botox® and soft-tissue fillers are poised to see huge growth in the market. Variations on Botox® using botulism toxin B rather than botulism toxin A are not yet approved by the FDA, but will provide longer-lasting results. Used in Europe since 1989, Artecoll may be the first permanent injection to treat wrinkles. The science behind it involves the injection of microscopic plastic beads suspended in collagen. Once the body absorbs the injected collagen, the tiny beads trigger the body to produce its own collagen, thus keeping the cycle of collagen production permanent. Every time the collagen depletes, the beads tell the body to produce more. Another form of collagen comes from a strange source: the discarded foreskins of infant boys after circumcision. CosmoDerm and Cosmo-Plast use the collagen-producing cells found in newborn foreskins, which are then replicated for use in cosmetic injections. Like the bovine collagen commonly used to treat wrinkles today, these products are eventually reabsorbed by the body and require another treatment three to six months later. CosmoDerm and Cosmo-Plast were both approved by the FDA for use on March 12, 2003.

The American Society for Aesthetic Plastic Surgeons (ASAPS) also predicts increases in bariatric and post-bariatric surgery. Used mainly for weight loss in morbidly obese people (more than 100 pounds overweight), bariatric surgery consists of either Lap-band surgery or stomach stapling, which reduce the size of the stomach and restrict how much food a patient can consume. Bariatric surgery also includes large-volume liposuction. After such procedures, patients are often left with massive amounts of loose skin. Full bodylift procedures remove the excess skin and reshape the patient's body in proportion to his or her new weight. In the face of an aging population that wants to hide evidence of its true years, cosmetic hand surgery is also expected to gain in popularity.

Along the lines of more is better, faster is also a priority. Lunchtime or quickie cosmetic procedures take minimal time, and the recovery time is a matter of hours rather than weeks. According to statistics from the American Society of Plastic Surgeons, over seven million minimally invasive surgical procedures were performed in 2003. With the ongoing approval of injectables like Botox® and Restylene (used for lip

enhancement), non-surgical cosmetic procedures will continue to see rapid growth.

Demand for plastic surgery has doubled and
even tripled in recent years. The stigma of plastic
surgery is vanishing as baby boomers erase their
wrinkles, younger people surgically improve what
nature gave them, and more celebrities openly
discuss their cosmetic improvements. More men
than ever before are also seeking out cosmetic
procedures such as skin resurfacing through microdermabrasion. Plastic surgery is becoming
one of many methods of looking and feeling one's
best, and surgeons are being added to a person's
support staff of aestheticians, hairdressers, fashion consultants, and personal trainers. But unlike
with fashion, plastic surgery trends are more difficult to drop when they become passé. Trendy
surgeries, such as buttock implants to emulate
the bodacious rear ends of stars like Jennifer
Lopez and Beyoncé Knowles, will inevitably fall
out of favor. Many surgeons refuse to perform
buttock implants based on the rationale that the

trend will pass and be replaced by the next body part du jour. Whatever the newest trends, it's likely that surgery-crazed consumers will have few qualms about going under the knife in order to acquire it.

The part of the population most affected by trends—teenagers—are one of the fastest growing segments of the industry. Rhinoplasty is the most common cosmetic operation for teenagers and has been for years. But now doctors are performing an increasing number of procedures such as breast implants, liposuction, and tummy tucks on girls as young as 14. In 2003, there were 11,326 breast enlargement procedures done on women 18 and under, representing 4 percent of the total number of breast augmentations performed in the U.S. From 2002 to 2003, according to the American Society for Aesthetic Plastic Surgery, the number of girls 18 and younger who got breast implants nearly tripled from 3,872 to 11,326. Breast implants have even become a popular high school graduation gift.

There are some frightening trends that could create significant problems if they continue unabated. The rapid growth of cosmetic surgery in the recent past shows no sign of slowing down. The exploding demand could see the emergence of more uncertified doctors wanting a share of the financial benefits of elective surgery. Uncertified doctors and dentists assume they can do procedures such as liposuction or one of the most challenging and subtle procedures, the nose job, with minimal or no training. Physicians are lying about credentials, concealing malpractice claims, and undermining the business of cosmetic surgery with bad practices. The demand of the market has already overtaken the controls set up by government medical licensing boards and professional certification organizations.

After the silicone-gel breast implant debacle and the scourge of uncertified and unregulated plastic surgery, the best-case scenario is increased government controls in the United

States. In 18 states, legislation battles rage over who is permitted to perform plastic surgery; 16 states already allow dental surgeons to perform plastic surgery. As the demand for multiple procedures increases and the injuries and deaths increase along with it, governments will have no choice but to become more involved in plastic surgery.

North American society and its pursuit of ageless perfection have reached new extremes with reality makeover TV shows. The general population is already clambering for the same drastic results shown on television. Multiple procedure surgeries are on the rise and show no signs of slowing despite their serious risks. The shows' use of computer imaging has now reached the mainstream and will become an important part of plastic surgeons' marketing plans. Computer imaging allows patients to see what they will look like after various procedures such as facelifts, breast augmentations, and liposuction. The power of suggestion can be intense in these situations, as patients see just how "perfect" they can become.

But some of the changes are intangible and unpredictable, and a change in appearance can have more ramifications than many people realize. Forty-five year old Susan Robinson was an average woman. Over the years her blonde hair had faded and begun to turn grey. She dyed it at home, and rarely did anything to pamper herself. Her teeth were crooked, and wrinkles had begun to gather around her eyes and mouth. Her stressful job as a social worker had also taken its toll, and she felt and looked drained. Even her social life was affected by her diminishing self-esteem.

Susan's teenage daughter Molly urged her to enter into an Ultimate Makeover contest sponsored by the Advanced Aesthetics Institute (AAI) of Palm Beach, Florida. The Institute offered aesthetic services from manicures and haircuts to complete plastic surgery. They held the event to showcase their services: a kind of real-life infomercial.

Much to her surprise, Susan won the contest, and ABC News picked up on her story. She arrived at the AAI where computer imaging was used to calculate Susan's "facial symmetry," and the clinic's technicians determined how an aesthetically improved version of herself would look. For Susan the change would involve a brow lift, eye job, chin implant, dental veneers, Botox®, permanent makeup, a breast lift and implants, tummy tuck, liposuction, a new haircut, and highlights.

Susan was excited about the makeover, but it was already influencing her life in subtle ways. First, she was hesitant to tell her husband, Guido Mayorga, about the makeover. The makeover was scheduled during the three weeks that the couple was to visit Ecuador, where Guido was born. On top of that, Guido's first wife had undergone plastic surgery in the Dominican Republic, and experienced major problems as a result. "What about if something goes wrong?" he asked news reporters.

Susan's first surgery was a five-hour brow lift, and afterward her confidence appeared to have had a lift as well. "This is the boldest thing I've ever done," she said. "That's so exciting." A few days later, she had another operation for her breasts, tummy tuck, and liposuction. People began treating her differently. She said people were more interested in her, that she was meeting "real friends." Her transformation continued with Botox® injections, painful cosmetic dentistry, and tattooed permanent makeup on her lips and eyebrows. The finishing touches were her new very blonde hairstyle, new clothes, and a style consultant who taught her how to walk and stand with better posture. She made her debut in a slinky long black dress with a plunging neckline. Her blue eyes sparkled and newly white teeth shone. The crowd clapped. Her daughter Molly cried. Guido was afraid she looked too good.

Just over two months after her transformation, Susan Robinson told ABC reporters that her husband seemed distant and wasn't touching her as much as before. He found that her facial expressions had changed. He said that he used to see her mother come through in her face, but since her surgeries, she wasn't there anymore. "I think we are still fine," Susan said at the time. "I mean, we know we love each other."

A year later, a follow-up article revealed that the two had begun divorce proceedings, and Mayorga was shattered by the breakup. "Susan's brain was changed," he told ABC. "Not just her body." The new and improved Susan? She had never felt or looked better, and although she won the contest, Susan Robinson paid a steep price for her new looks.

A Plastic Surgery Timeline

600 BC
Hindu author Sushruta describes nose reconstruction

695 AD
Emperor Justinian II's nose is amputated and his power usurped. He receives a reconstruction, and returns to power in 10 years

1200s Pope Innocent III prohibits all surgical procedures

1570 Leonardo Fioravanti reports first successful skin graft

1794 Account of a nose reconstruction in India published in a British magazine brings plastic surgery to England

1818 German surgeon Carl Von Graefe publishes *Rhinoplastik*. First use of word "plastic," derived from the Greek word *plastikos* meaning "to mold" or "to give form"

1890s Dr. Robert Gersuny uses paraffin wax injections for breast augmentation

1891 American John Roe performs nose surgery for cosmetic purposes

1914–1918
Sir Harold Gillies performs reconstructive surgery on more than 5,000 wounded soldiers

1921 French surgeon Charles Dujarrier attempts to remove fat from a dancer's leg resulting in infection and amputation

1924 First formal training program and fellowship in plastic surgery at Johns Hopkins University

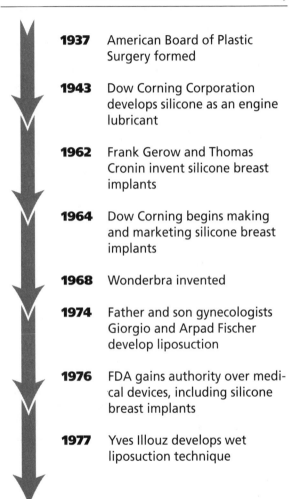

1937 American Board of Plastic Surgery formed

1943 Dow Corning Corporation develops silicone as an engine lubricant

1962 Frank Gerow and Thomas Cronin invent silicone breast implants

1964 Dow Corning begins making and marketing silicone breast implants

1968 Wonderbra invented

1974 Father and son gynecologists Giorgio and Arpad Fischer develop liposuction

1976 FDA gains authority over medical devices, including silicone breast implants

1977 Yves Illouz develops wet liposuction technique

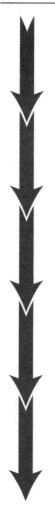

1987   American dermatologist
Jeffery Klein invents
tumescent liposuction

Ophthalmologist Jean
Carruthers discovers
cosmetic uses of Botox®

1990   *Face To Face With Connie
Chung* sparks silicone breast
implant inquest

1992   Silicone implants taken off the
market

1998   Dow Corning settles lawsuit for
$3.2 billion payable to 170,000
women

1999   Physicians in Florida required
to report events including
patient deaths and emergency
transfers to hospitals occurring
during office-based procedures

2000   U.S. Department of Health
finds no evidence that silicone
implants cause autoimmune
disease

2001 State of Florida establishes 90-day ban on procedures requiring general anesthesia performed in office setting

2002 FDA approves Botox® (botulinum toxin A)

First season of *Extreme Makeover* airs

2003 Dutch study reveals that women with breast implants are three times more likely to commit suicide than general public

Chinese beauty queen Yang Yuan is barred from entering a beauty pageant when organizers discover she had extensive plastic surgery

2004 New Jersey institutes six percent sales tax on cosmetic surgery procedures

"Miss Plastic Surgery" pageant held in Beijing, China

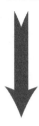

2004   State of Florida sets 90-day
           ban on performing liposuction
           and tummy tuck together

2005   FDA approves use of Mentor
           Corp's silicone-gel implant

Amazing Facts and Figures

American Statistics

• According to the American Society of Plastic Surgeons, more than 250,000 women had breast augmentation surgery in 2003. More than 68,000 women chose breast reconstruction following a mastectomy or injury.

• Breast augmentation increased 657 percent from 1992 to 2003, and breast reconstruction procedures increased by 131 percent.

• There were 11.9 million cosmetic procedures in the U.S. in 2004. That represents a 44 percent increase over the previous year. (American Society for Aesthetic Plastic Surgery)

• In the U.S., the number of surgical cosmetic procedures increased 17 percent and the number of non-surgical procedures increased 51 percent from 2003 to 2004. The most frequently performed non-surgical procedure was Botox® injection and the most popular surgical procedure was liposuction.

Plastic Surgery Patients By Age

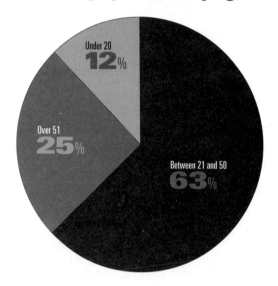

- Women accounted for 90 percent of all cosmetic procedures performed in the U.S. in 2004. The number of surgical and non-surgical procedures performed on women was nearly 10.7 million.

- American men had 1.2 million cosmetic procedures throughout 2004, which was up by 8 percent over 2003. More men had non-surgical procedures, including Botox® and laser hair removal, than surgical procedures.

Top Surgical and Non-Surgical Cosmetic Procedures, 2004

Surgical	# of procedures
Liposuction	478,251
Breast augmentation	334,052
Eyelid surgery	290,343
Rhinoplasty	166,187
Facelift	157,061
Non-surgical	
Botox	2,837,346
Laser hair removal	1,411,899
Chemical peel	1,110,401
Microdermabrasion	1,098,316
Lip Enhancement	882,469

- Just over 46 percent of cosmetic procedures in 2004 were performed in office-based facilities; 29.1 percent were done in freestanding surgicenters; and 24.4 percent were performed in hospitals.

- Americans spent just under $12.5 billion on cosmetic procedures in 2004; $7.7 billion of that was spent on surgical procedures and $4.7 billion was for non-surgical procedures.

Surgical Procedures	US	CDN
Breast augmentation	$3,373	$6,000
Breast lift	$3,718	$6,000
Buttock lift	$3,630	$2,500–8,000
Cheek implant	$1,854	$3,500
Chin augmentation	$1,512	$2,500
Dermabrasion	$866	n/a
Eyelid surgery	$2,523	$5,000
Facelift	$4,822	$8,000
Forehead lift	$2,400	$4,000
Liposuction	$2,223	$2,000
Lower body lift	$6,425	$8,000
Nose reshaping	$3,332	$4,000
Tummy tuck	$4,505	$5,000
Upper arm lift	$3,106	$2,000–5,000
Non-surgical Procedures		
Botox	$376	$500
Cellulite treatment	$127	n/a
Chemical peel	$607	$1,000–5,000
Laser hair removal	$428	$200–2,000
Laser skin resurfacing	$2,117	$4,000
Microdermabrasion	$173	$100–200
Lip Enhancement using Hyaluronic acid	$539	n/a

Sources: American Society of Plastic Surgeons, average fees 2004. Average Canadian fees 2003

Canadian Statistics (from Medicard)

• In 2003, there were over 302,000 surgical and non-surgical cosmetic enhancements performed in Canada. This is an increase of nearly 60,000 procedures, or 24.6 percent from 2002.

• Canadians spent more than $5 billion on cosmetic procedures in 2003.

• In 2003, liposuction procedures increased by 16 percent from 2002 reaching 24,337, which is 24 percent of the surgical market in Canada.

• The number of patients having non-surgical facelift procedures grew dramatically in 2003 to 17,628 patients.

• Canadian women are seeking 85.5 percent of all cosmetic enhancement procedures; the most popular are liposuction, breast augmentation, and non-surgical facelift. Men most often seek liposuction, rhinoplasty, and eye lifts.

• The number of breast implant procedures rose 17 percent to16,973 in 2003.

• Ontario accounts for 42 percent of cosmetic procedures performed in Canada, followed by British Columbia at 26 percent and Alberta with 11 percent.

International Statistics

• In 2003, the world witnessed a 20 percent increase in the overall number of plastic surgeries performed.

• The 10 countries performing the most plastic surgeries account for 68 percent of the world's total procedures. The top five countries are all located on the American continents: USA, Mexico, Brazil, Canada, and Argentina. These 5 countries account for 47 percent of the procedures performed worldwide. Europe comes next, with Spain, France, and Germany totaling 14 percent. Japan and South Africa follow with 7 percent of the total procedures.

• The world percentage of patients who seek aesthetic surgery is 88 percent female and 12 percent male.

• Percent of patients under 21 years by country
    #1 South Africa: 45.71 percent
    #7 Canada 17.92 percent
    #23 United States 6.98 percent

What Others Say

"For actresses, their looks are their jobs. It's not an issue of vanity. It's a necessity."

Cosmetic dermatologist Dr. Anna Guanche

"Botox® freaks me out."

Actress Cameron Diaz

"Aging is the field of the future."

Manhattan dermatologist and plastic surgeon Dr. Douglas Altcheck

"It's the difference between a Hyundai and a BMW."

Dr. Deborah Bash, plastic surgeon, on saline versus silicone breast implants

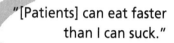

"[Patients] can eat faster
than I can suck."

*Dr. Gerald Pitman, one of the
top liposuctionists in the U.S.*

"I wish I had a twin, so I could know what
I'd look like without plastic surgery."

Joan Rivers

"I'm 100 percent, all-natural
American chick right now."

*Catherine Hickland, former "One Life
to Live" soap star, who went in for a
minor breast lift, was given breast
implants without her consent, and
lived with them for several years.
Eventually, she got them removed and
had another breast lift surgery.*

"I haven't frowned since 1987."

Jean Carruthers, Botox® inventor

"A strengthening economy means that people are more willing to invest in the things that improve their quality of life. Feeling good about the way they look is high on the list of priorities for many Americans."

Former ASAPS President Robert Bernard, MD

"This is a major surgical procedure, not a hairdo."

Adam Searle, president of the British Association of Aesthetic Plastic Surgery (BAAPS)

"Why grow old gracefully when you have the technology to prevent it?"

TV star Nicole Richie

"The issue of untrained or inadequately trained practitioners, some of whom are not medical doctors, performing cosmetic plastic surgery is an extremely serious patient safety concern."

Los Angeles plastic surgeon and ASAPS former President Peter B. Fodor, MD.

I was told that it wasn't even possible, as there are three rules in cosmetic surgery: 1) You can't make a plain person attractive; 2) You can't change bone structure; 3) You can't take more than 10 years off a face. I broke all three rules and set a world record.

Cindy Jackson, "Living Barbie"

"I'd have a facelift. Absolutely! [But] there are some women who have gone way too far."

Actress Jennifer Aniston

Bibliography

Andrews, Michelle. "Vacation makeovers." *U.S. News & World Report*, 00415537, 1/19/2004, Vol. 136, Issue 2.

Adato, Allison, Adrienne Bard, Cary Cardwell, Maureen Harrington, Andrea Orr, Tracie Powell, Charlotte Triggs, Jennifer Wulff. "Plastic Surgery South of the Border: Is It Safe?" *People*, 00937673, 6/20/2005, Vol. 63, Issue 24.

Adato, Allison, Susan Schneider Simison, and Melody Simmons. "The Return of Silicone?" *People*, 00937673, 5/2/2005, Vol. 63, Issue 17.

Bamji, A. "Gillies: an historical vignette." *Trauma*, 1999, Vol. 1 Issue 3, p267, 3p, 2bw.

Bellafante, Ginia and Elaine Shannon. "Death by Makeover," *TIME Australia*, 07/21/97 Issue

29, p29, 1p, 1c, 1bw.

Boodman, Sandra G. "For More Teenage Girls, Adult Plastic Surgery," *Washington Post.* Tuesday, October 26, 2004; Page A01.

Brant, Martha and John Barry. "Liposuctioned to death." *Newsweek*, 07/21/97, Vol. 130 Issue 3, p43, 1p, 1c.

"Breast Implant Patient Guilty in Surgeon's Death," *Los Angeles Times.* Los Angeles, Calif.: Feb 12, 1999. pg. 26.

Canadian Medical Association Journal, 10/19/99, Vol. 161, Issue 8, p1028, 2p.

Corcoran Flynn, Timothy, MD, William P. Coleman III, MD, Lawrence M. Field, MD, Jeffrey A. Klein, MD, and C. William Hanke, MD. "History of Liposuction." *Dermatologic Surgery.* 26 (6), 515-520, June 2000.

Daane S.P. and W.B. Rockwell. "Analysis of methods for reporting severe and mortal liposuction complications." *Aesthetic Plastic Surgery.* Volume 23 (5), 1999, p 303-306.

Eisenberg, David M., Ronald C. Kessler, Cindy Foster, Frances E. Norlock, David R. Calkins, Thomas L. Delbanco. "Unconventional Medicine in the United States—Prevalence, Costs, and Patterns of Use," *The New England Journal of Medicine.* January 28, 1993, Vol. 328, No. 4.

Fleisher, Lee A. M.D., Gerard F. Anderson Ph.D., "Perioperative Risk: How Can We Study the Influence of Provider Characteristics?" *Anesthesiology,* Volume 96(5), May 2002, pp 1039-1041.

Fox, Isadora. "The Perfect Margaret Trigg," *New York Magazine,* May 3, 2004.

Gardner Jr., Ralph. "Looks to Die For," *New York Magazine,* February 16, 2004.

Green, Michelle and Natasha Stoynoff. "First Wives Club author Olivia Goldsmith dies during cosmetic surgery," *People*, 00937673, 2/2/2004, Vol. 61, Issue 4.

Hayden, Maureen. "The rise and fall of Wally Zollman," *Indianapolis Monthly*, Feb2004, Vol. 27 Issue 7, p134, 7p, 3c.

Iverson, Ronald E., M.D., Dennis J. Lynch, M.D., and the ASPS Committee on Patient Safety. "Practice Advisory on Liposuction," Pleasanton, Calif. Vol. 113, No. 5 / PRACTICE ADVISORY ON LIPOSUCTION, pg 1478–1490.

Knepper v. Dex Media, Inc., Or., Multnomah County Cir. Ct., No. 9903-02495, Feb. 14, 2005.

Kolesnikov-Jessop, Sonia. "Holiday Enhancements," *Newsweek (Atlantic Edition)*, 01637053, 3/14/2005, Vol. 145, Issue 11.

Leslie, Colin. "The private clinic debate," Medical Post Online Edition, May 09, 2000, Volume 36 Issue 18.

Lewis, Cynthia. "Going Plastic in Costa Rica." Antioch Review, Winter 2005, Vol. 63 Issue 1, p6, 17p.

Lloyd Billingsley, Kenneth. "Affirmative Action in Action: Doctor No," FrontPageMagazine.com, September 1, 1997.http://www.frontpagemag.com/Articles/ReadArticle.asp?ID=3425

McInture, Mike and Jack Dolan. "Dangerous Doctors." *The Hartford Courant* online edition, April 30, 2000. http://www.courant.com/news/specials/hc-story-npdb1,0,5390175.story

New Scientist, 10/30/2004, Vol. 184 Issue 2471, p.54, 3p.

"Numbers," *TIME*, 0040781X, 4/18/2005, Vol. 165, Issue 16.

"Operating Under the Radar." *People*, 00937673, 6/20/2005, Vol. 63, Issue 24.

"Plastic surgeons affected by economy, paid on production," *Physician Compensation Report.* Oct 2002.

"Plastic Surgical Techniques in the Fifteenth Century by Serafeddin Sabuncuoglu," *Plastic & Reconstructive Surgery.* 99(6):1775-1779, May 1997, Teoman Dogan M.D.; Mehmet Bayramicli M.D.; Ayhan Numanoglu M.D.

Prevention, Nov 2003, Vol. 55, Issue 11, p146, 2p.

Querna, Elizabeth. "Health Risk or a Woman's Choice?" *U.S. News & World Report*, 00415537, 4/25/2005, Vol. 138, Issue 15.

Sissell, Kara. "Dow Corning Emerges from Bankruptcy." *Chemical Week*, 0009272X, 6/9/2004, Vol. 166, Issue 19.

Solis, Dianne. "Mexico's most-powerful drug lord dies following extensive plastic surgery," *Wall Street Journal—Eastern Edition*, 07/07/97, Vol. 230 Issue 4, pA14.

Toledano, Jessica. "Legislature Eyes Increased Regulation of Plastic Surgery," *Orange County Business Journal.* 10517480, 02/22/99, Vol. 28, Issue 8.

Tran, Tini. "A Look Back: Challenge and Change in Orange County From El Toro to El Nino, a Stormy Year." *Los Angeles Times* (Orange County), Sunday, January 4, 1998.

Wellace, Amy. "Face-off: the confounding case of Marchioni v. Keyes," *Los Angeles Magazine.* Sept, 2003.

Yoho, R.A. *et al.* "Review of the liposuction, abdominoplasty, and face-lift mortality and morbidity risk literature," *Dermatological Surgery*, July 2005, Volume 31 (7 Pt 1), p 733–43.

Acknowledgments

Several people were invaluable in their assistance and direction on this project. Thank you to Dr. Earl Campbell and Dr. Dale Birdsell for their professional grace and knowledge. Thank you to Drs. Allan and Charlotte Jones, in more ways than I can ever innumerate. Thanks also to Kimberly and Angela Jones for keeping me sane. Many thanks to my friends for tolerating my non-stop cocktail party stories of botched plastic surgery, and my general obsession during the writing of this book. And, as always, thank you to Stephen Hutchings and Kara Turner for their enthusiasm and vision.

Photo credits

Cover: Getty Images; Alamy Images (A30480): page 8; AP Photos: pages 9 (John Hayes); 10 (East Valley Tribune, Darryl Webb), 11 (York Daily Record/Sunday News, Jason Plotkin), 12 (Handout), 13 (John Hayes).

LATE-BREAKING
AMAZING STORIES™

IDENTITY THEFT

The scary new crime that targets all of us
by Rennay Craats

www.amazingstoriesbooks.com